REDISCOVER
YOUR
ATHLETE WITHIN

REDISCOVER YOUR ATHLETE WITHIN

A practical 10-step process to get you moving and keep you moving, for the rest of your life

Dr Brett Lillie

with Lisa Lillie

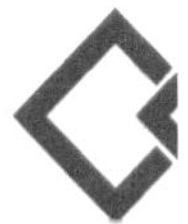

'IF WE WERE
MEANT TO STAY
IN ONE PLACE,
WE WOULD HAVE
ROOTS INSTEAD
OF FEET.'

—

RACHEL WOLCHIN

WHAT OTHERS SAY ABOUT DR BRETT AND
REDISCOVER YOUR ATHLETE WITHIN

'Ah – it's about time! A simple, eloquent, fast-paced, step-by-step guide that shows you how to change your thinking so you can change your mind and let go of past beliefs that limit who you are. Then, with the grace of a professional athlete, Dr Lillie provides the what to do to put your body in motion. The end result, better health, more and longer mobility and increased happiness. I'd say that is soooo cool!'

**Dr Larry Markson, Author of *Talking to Yourself is Not Crazy*,
The Cabin Experience**

'What an inspiring book to get you to appreciate the Athlete Within. His stories of his patients and their journey really gets you to think… "what's holding me back?" Brett, you got me to start making changes in my life thanks to your book.'

**Dr Mayoor Patel
Author of *Sleep Apnea Hurts – the cure doesn't have to* and *Take a Bite out of Pain***

'Brett's energy and passion really come through. I read the book on a plane trip from San Diego to Boston and I couldn't put it down. It was the perfect message for me to revive my energy. I want the best me as I close in on 70.'

**Dr Steven Olmos
Founder of the TMJ & Sleep Therapy Centres**

'This book made me reflect internally about whether I've been doing a good enough job at making the most of me, particularly the physical me. How much better condition could I be in? I'll be 67 shortly – I think I should resume training. If, like most, you have let your physical condition slip, you may want to consult the excuses list in this book and then embrace the strategies suggested to do something about it.'

Dr John I. Kelly DC FACC FICC

'Brett has an unmatched passion for physical wellbeing. I know because I spent 15 years attending his Sydney clinic. Brett has been an essential ingredient in ensuring my athletic performance at 60 is superior to that of when I was 40. Sounds unbelievable but it's true. The man works miracles … I have seen them with my own eyes.'

Craig Anderson
Executive Director, Princeton

'Purely delightful reading.'

Dr Catherine Norton
CEO and Director, Heal with Laser

'Brett makes you see things in a different way, challenges your thinking and is incredibly curious. A conversation with him is always interesting and rarely goes as you expect.'

Lucas Kohlenberg & Yolande Nyss

'Brett has fundamentally changed how I think about rehabilitation and recovery.'

Ben Matthews

'What an eye-opening approach to finding not only my inner athlete, but inner strength and confidence and love for self. The Athlete Within was able to capture and explain my darkest moments and turned them into actionable steps.'

Dr Andrea Sargent DC (Canada)

'Brett has a sixth sense when it comes to pain and rehabilitation. He always shares his wisdom with patience, generosity and lots of encouragement!'

Jill Fulcher

'What an excellent book. It certainly made me review the steps I have taken! It is very helpful for us all to ensure we keep moving and really think how we want to be at 80 or 90.'

Judy Snowdon
Pilates and DNS instructor

'We owe our awareness and wellness to Brett. He is not just hands on but "mind on".'

Rebecca and Simon Turner

'If there is someone who knows what they're talking about – it's Brett! He is so knowledgeable and has a knack for educating his clients so they want to continue working on themselves. Thank you Brett for inspiring us to be the best we can be.'

Angela Garcia

'This book is a personal health booster. It will re-energise the chronically ill and unfit. It will also tune up the amateur or professional athlete. Start at the beginning and go to the end, or dip in at the points where you need help now: this book will be useful however you choose to read it.'

Julie Garland McLellan
CEO of The Director's Dilemma

'Brett is not your ordinary chiropractor, and this is not your ordinary "wellbeing" book. As I flipped each page, I could see Brett's smiling face right there, coming along for the ride (as he aptly describes it) to encourage me not only to find my Athlete Within but also to help me maintain it. A great concept cleverly narrated.'

Damien Roberts

DEDICATION

To the love of my life Lisa,
for your never-ending ability to live life and press my buttons

To my five beautiful children
Amber, Alexander, Alexandra, Scarlett and Ryder

To my mum
for your love through my thick and thin

To Jas – you've got this

To those of you who know
deep inside
there is an athlete within
waiting to get out

To you

First published in 2023 by Dr Brett Lillie

A catalogue entry for this book is available from the National Library of Australia.

ISBN: 978-1-922764-83-6

Book production and text design by Publish Central
Cover design by Julia Kuris
Back cover photo by Jason Malouin

Disclaimer: The material in this publication is of the nature of general comment only, and does not represent professional advice. It is not intended to provide specific guidance for particular circumstances and it should not be relied on as the basis for any decision to take action or not take action on any matter which it covers. Readers should obtain professional advice where appropriate, before making any such decision. To the maximum extent permitted by law, the author and publisher disclaim all responsibility and liability to any person, arising directly or indirectly from any person taking or not taking action based on the information in this publication.

CONTENTS

INTRODUCTION

HOW I DISCOVERED THE ATHLETE WITHIN

I have come to believe inside every one of us there's an Athlete Within, an athletic element, an evolutionary and ancient drive to want to move, an urge to be more. You only have to look at a child excited on a swing in a park to be taken right back to a time in your own past when you were that little kid, full of energy, vibrant with life, wanting to move and explore just because it was fun.

Truth is, you may not have felt like this for a very long time. Life just happens. It's busy, it's messy, it's full on. But life is also beautiful, full of hope and possibilities. In fact, it doesn't mean that you're stuck and can't experience that amazing feeling again. I believe inside every one of us there's an athlete that never goes away, you just need a process to find your way back to rediscover it. And you can do that, right now, at any age, on your terms. This book is your process.

Your Athlete Within is waiting, it's ready for you, it's up to you now to find it and give it life and I know you can. I believe you can.

As a chiropractor, you get to know people and understand where they are at. You quietly enter their lives and you become part of their team. As they get to know you, they begin to share more and more about themselves. And it's their stories that have been some of my greatest teachers, inspirations and sources of pride. Treating them, I constantly improved myself and became better at what I do, but I also came to understand their journeys, how they were putting the pieces of their puzzles together to make meaning of their life. Their worries, their angsts, their pain. Their hopes, their dreams, their visions.

When I was 26 I was in a motorbike accident. I was always very cautious on two wheels but that afternoon it was raining and the lady who accidentally cut in front and hit me simply didn't see me. I broke my right shoulder, and my collar bone had pretty much become a knife precariously situated right next to the brachial plexus, which is nothing other than the nerve supply to the arm. If cut, I would have been left with a loosely hanging limb.

At the time I was in the second-last year of my Chiropractic Master's Degree, so I took all I had learnt up to that point and diligently applied it to my own recovery. Within months I had regained good control and stability of my right arm and by all standards felt I was back to normal.

A few years went by and all was falling nicely into place. A happy marriage, a bigger clinic, more patients, more knowledge and confidence. Except, I started to experience pain along the left side of my body, particularly in my neck. At first the pain only occurred occasionally, but then it became more frequent and began impacting my practice. With time, the pain was a daily occurrence that drained me and left me exhausted. My life as I knew it was drifting, my career was being disrupted and I was struggling to find a solution.

I had always been a very curious learner. Whenever an answer didn't quite fit a question or a solution wasn't as effective as I had hoped, I would explore other avenues and question my understanding of the world. The pain I was experiencing was no different: there had to be a reason. And so, after exhausting all usual avenues, I knew I had to follow my gut and continue searching, studying and immersing myself in the world of other disciplines.

That's when I started walking other paths.

In Prague I studied under Dr Karel Lewit, pioneer of modern diagnostics and treatment of musculoskeletal disorders. Simply put, he was the Yoda of rehabilitation. And just like the great Jedi master, he too challenged my approach and pushed me to think independently and in a way that forced deeper understanding. It was ultimately Dr Pavel Kolar – another freakishly good younger Jedi master – who had the biggest influence on me and provided answers that fit my questions. He taught me to look at the way my patients moved and compare them against ideal patterns to identify issues and discrepancies. It was no longer just about 'where it hurts' but also about 'how it moves' and 'why it hurts'.

At the same time I was jumping across another ocean and landed in the US where Dr Steven Olmos, an orofacial specialist who took lateral thinking to a whole new level, was deep into studying chronic pain and everything that went with it. I was now entering the world of sleep medicine and pathological ageing.

At that point I made a promise to myself that I would always look at the bigger picture, not just where the problem seemed to be. I would always be curious and continue to expand my understanding of the human body and mind. That's where the thinking and approach behind the Athlete Within had its roots.

It was however years later in the clinic that I started to form the belief that inside every one of us is an athlete, someone with a dream of being able to do more, be more and become more.

In my clinic I was seeing the effects a sedentary life had on my clients. Injecting movement back into their lives as a way of reconnecting to what made them happy often meant they could overcome pain (and overcome their own story) and become who they wanted to be. I could see that they had different starting points but ended up following a specific path to achieve their goals. They were invested emotionally and physically, and – even if each journey was individual – the steps to become their Athlete Within were the same.

I had to follow those very steps back in 2013 when, at 44 years of age and four days before Christmas, my life turned upside down.

I had known something was wrong, but the stress of a prolonged divorce while running a busy clinic had blurred my thinking, and even the doctors hadn't been able to put their finger on what was happening. I showed up at Emergency at 3 am. Something was just *wrong*, and it's then that I knew I had to stop and really make sense of it all. And in an instant my life didn't just change, it flipped on its head with a shattering diagnosis.

The reality of walking into a hospital mere days before Christmas meant doctors and nurses were working at reduced shifts. MRIs were done first thing in the morning, colonoscopies at 11 pm. It was hours of waiting, worrying, not knowing, and then going into rooms to be tested and prodded, feeling uncomfortable the whole time. My surgeon delivered the news: it was colon cancer, and the prognosis was three months.

I had to absorb the enormity of the moment.

The next day, I had family near my bed and the children were running around. Looking up from my recumbent position, I saw everything in slow motion and I knew I had to go inside and look at myself. I had spent so much of my life putting other people ahead of me, following what I thought was right – now it was my ultimate decision. Life was closing one door on me but I saw this as a second chance, my act two. Another door was opening, and I stepped through.

Boxing Day was surgery, first thing in the morning. The process had begun, and so had the process in my head. I wasn't sure exactly how, but I had to let go to move on, to reach new ground. Internal determination now set in, and life was never going to be the same.

It was here I truly learned how to block out noise and distraction to follow my own story, my own desires, my true me. I had to revisit principles I shared with my clients to see if they rang true for me. I was meditating and visualising my future, I was 'staying in my own lane' (one of my favourite principles). I wasn't living according to the scoreboard and I was following what worked for me. I embraced my pace and started to embody the principle of 'slow burn'. I was living the lessons I taught for so many years, feeling them in my mind and my body. I knew then that I could find me again and move into a better, improved version. One that had no stress and no regrets. A version of me that prioritised my values and an active lifestyle. I wanted love, fun, adventure, and I had clarity. I was moving forward and away from my illness. I was aligning with my Athlete Within.

I was just about to turn 50. Professor Stuart McGill, one of the world-leading experts in back pain and none other than my absolute hero, was in Australia to give his final lecture – he was on his retirement tour. I was there, front row. During one of the lunch breaks the other students went off to get some food and I found myself sharing a table with Professor McGill. It was just us, and I was nervous. We started chatting. We exchanged thoughts and ideas. We discussed functional training, what he was doing to keep in shape, and the importance of recovery. Then, out of the blue, he said to me: 'I train harder and I'm stronger now at the age of 78 than when I was 50 years old.'

You can imagine the questions that started going through my head: *What just happened? How is that possible? What does he mean? How does he do it? But also: Ohhhh noooo, I'm nearly 50 … what am I going to do? Am I doomed? It can't be …* After that simple revelation, he sprang out of his chair and ran back to the lecture theatre.

At the end of the seminar I went home to my family, and after helping my wife put the kids to bed, I found some quiet time to take a breath, collect my thoughts and think about what had happened just a few hours earlier. It all made sense. Professor McGill embodied my idea of the Athlete Within. I knew how to rediscover the Athlete Within. It was time for me to put pen to paper (or fingers to the keyboard).

And that is how this book came about.

Rediscovering your athlete is something you carry with you forever. As you grow and you enter new decades, your priorities and needs change too. And to be true to your wants and desires, you have to make changes that can be small but also quite radical.

I am currently putting the finishing touches on this book from a small office in Hobart, Tasmania. How I got here, having lived in Sydney all my life? My Athlete Within (and that of my wife) implored me to slow down and adjust the pace, to reconnect with nature and find a way of life that was closer to my truth. This is why you can often find me running up the trail of a ridiculously steep hill (through the bush) on my way to collect the kids from school. Who knows what my Athlete Within has in store for me next?

I cannot wait to hear your story. To help you along your journey of rediscovery and celebrate the moments. To meet you and your new you.

HOW TO GET THE MOST OUT OF THIS BOOK

Rediscover Your Athlete Within is designed to help you get off the couch and embrace a more active life. It's definitely a journey and only you can decide the destination, how far or simply where you want to go. We start from way back with your old you, when you were a kid, remembering what you were good at, what you loved, what you were naturally drawn to, all the way to reconnecting with that part of you now and becoming your true you.

This book is intended to be for everyone; it is inclusive at its core. I hope to inspire you, through practical steps that are within reach but far away enough to keep you going. This process is designed to challenge you to be a little bit more *you*, a little bit better, and a little bit more athletic.

Here's how to get the most out of this book …

1. Flick through the book

Well, you got this far, it's now time to be naughty and flick through the rest of the book. The aim is for you to have an idea about what's ahead and how it all fits together. Start getting into the groove of rediscovering your Athlete Within. Get a feel for what's coming before you go back to the start and dive in.

2. Follow the sequence ... or not

This book has 10 steps that have been developed in a particular sequence that just works. Ideally you'd start from Step 1 and get to Step 10 in the order suggested. I find those who follow and stick to the process step by step in the right sequence are more likely to find success and really build from what they learn through the framework.

Ultimately though, I want you to be yourself. Your true self. And if you're inclined to jump around, take side steps and find inspiration your own way, please do so. My desire for you is to rediscover your Athlete Within and live your best life, one way or another.

3. Make time

This one sounds super hard, and we all know why. Finding time is often one of the biggest issues we encounter. But you have to make time to read the book. To explore each step. You have decided to invest in yourself so the best thing you can do is schedule ahead and book time in advance, just as you would a meeting or a Christmas party. This is your time and you need it to absorb the messages, the learnings and explore your Athlete Within.

4. Do it all

However you approach this book, I'd love you to complete all the steps. Why? This process has 10 steps for a really good reason. It touches on 10 aspects of your inner athlete. Some sections will speak to you more and some may not leave a massive mark, but they all have a purpose and they can all really help you be the best you can be.

You may pick the book up at different moments, and chances are you will take home something different or something new every time. That's the beauty of rediscovering the Athlete Within. It is about you, where you are and who you are right now.

5. Do it with intention

In each section you'll find some ideas, questions and exercises to help you rediscover your Athlete Within. Take a moment and give these challenges a go. As you move deeper into the process I'll help you find more purpose, meaning and even hope, but the journey starts with you. It's about allowing yourself to be on the path, not doing it perfectly. There is a downloadable workbook on our website that can help you go through these exercises. Head over to brettlillie.com to grab your free copy.

6. Stop and stare

We can all find inspiration everywhere, yet it is our own experiences that can offer the greatest wealth and greatest resource to tap into. If a thought, a memory, an experience resurfaces during the process, capture it. Stop and stare at the moment because it may be a message, the key to opening a deeper part of yourself or seeing the road ahead.

7. But I am not an athlete

Ahh ... my favourite excuse, along with all the stories of why we can't do it.

If you think you're not an athlete then this book *is definitely for you*.

Many things in life work but they don't necessarily make sense. Take the English language for example and all its beautiful rules. Did you know there are nine different ways to pronounce the letters 'ough'? It makes no sense.

In this book I am going to make you think about things differently, and that includes your version of what an athlete is. All I ask is that you keep an open mind and have fun along the way. Be surprised by your discoveries, inspired by the possibilities and amazed by what you're capable of.

WHAT IS THE ATHLETE WITHIN?

Now if I asked you to describe what an athlete is, I'm sure you would start thinking of someone who is super fit, sweaty and wearing sports clothes. People who are disciplined, pushing their body to the limit, for hours upon hours in gruelling training schedules, all leading up to a big event. Things like swimming, rugby, grand slam tennis or the big-ticket events like the Olympics. Platforms with serious elite competitors fighting it out. Right?

But let's talk a little about what being an athlete means to you. To do that we need to go back in time to visit some distant relatives.

There was a time when being a valued member of a village meant doing your bit, playing a role useful to the village as a whole. In most instances, your role was related to your physical capability. If you were strong, your job was to lift heavy things. But there were other factors that would influence your role. For example, if you had an innate understanding of nature and the environment, you could grow food. A highly valued role in any community.

In times of plenty a feast might be held to celebrate the harvest. Other villages would come to trade and share ideas. It would have been a time of opportunity, with people showing off their abilities, and in a way it was the beginning of sport. Competition would have evolved naturally, with people trying to best each other.

Of course this has morphed over thousands of years to the modern world where we have a very clear definition of what an athlete is. We follow sporting teams and sporting heroes, we have major events, even our children are encouraged to be athletes from the youngest of ages. Athlete, athlete, athlete …

Well, I see things a little differently.

What if an athlete is someone just actively being themselves, working towards a level that's in accordance with their own characteristic talents, abilities and nature? Where being active and in the right condition is also about being in tune with who you are. Where we are allowed to go through periods of intensity that reflect the seasons and stages of our lives. And at the same time not dropping the ball when the going gets tough. For the true athlete, movement becomes a way of life.

So, what I'm really trying to do here is get you to rethink what being an athlete means. This book is all about helping you rediscover your Athlete Within, but you get to choose what *your* athlete looks like. I'm not trying to turn you into an Olympic weightlifter or an ultra-marathon runner (unless you want to). I want to help you rediscover that wonderful energy and sense of fulfilment that comes from moving the way you used to, without overthinking it.

I watch my six-year-old twins play and they couldn't be more different. One is like a monkey – she is on from the moment she wakes, running and jumping everywhere until her head touches the pillow that night. The other is a turtle – she is slow to wake and harder to get to sleep. A little princess, she does not run, she only dances, everywhere, mostly ballet. Did we teach them any of this? No. It is their way, their nature. It just resonates and oozes out of them. Your athlete has been with you since the beginning. If you look back, you will see your athletic self rise to the surface.

Your Athlete Within could be a dancer, rock climber, walker, hiker, roller skater, dog walker, bike rider, volleyball player – it's a *very* long list. But remember, it's *your* Athlete Within. And it is most definitely tied in to the athlete you were as a kid.

This is the perfect place to ask you two questions:

· What is your current definition of being an athlete?
· If you rethink what being an athlete means to you, what does that look like?

Once we've defined what being an athlete means, and at the same time, redefined what you want your Athlete Within to look like, we can take the next step in this journey. Rediscovering your Athlete Within is not only about rediscovering the best things about your past but also how to keep refining where you are now, taking aim to a better future, a better you.

ARE YOU TALL ENOUGH FOR THIS RIDE?

My son was exceptionally tall for a 12-year-old. Having grown five centimetres in the last three months, he easily passed the required height for entry. He was standing in front of this insane, let's call it a 'roller-coaster', but it was clearly much more intense than a good old-fashioned roller-coaster. This thing would speed forward, come to a sudden halt, throw everyone this way and that, then hit reverse hard. He looked at this ride and then he looked at me. *Surely not,* I thought. But then he was young and full of bravado.

'Dad, can I go on this ride?'

The sign says if you are 'this' tall – that's the only requirement. In my head, I urgently ran through the list of reasons why not: you're too young? You just finished your lunch? Your mum will kill me? And then I shifted to his side of the fence; this might be his only opportunity to try a ride this intense at this age. If I say no, the rest of the day will be filled with regret, maybe even the rest of this week? The rest of this trip will have this cloud. I turned to him and – without showing my hesitation – said, 'Yes … let's do it together!'

You picked up this book, now you've got the ticket in your hand and you're about to go on your own roller-coaster ride. Chances are you *are* tall enough for this ride, but just in case you're worried, don't be, because I'm coming along with you.

This is the journey you are embarking on …

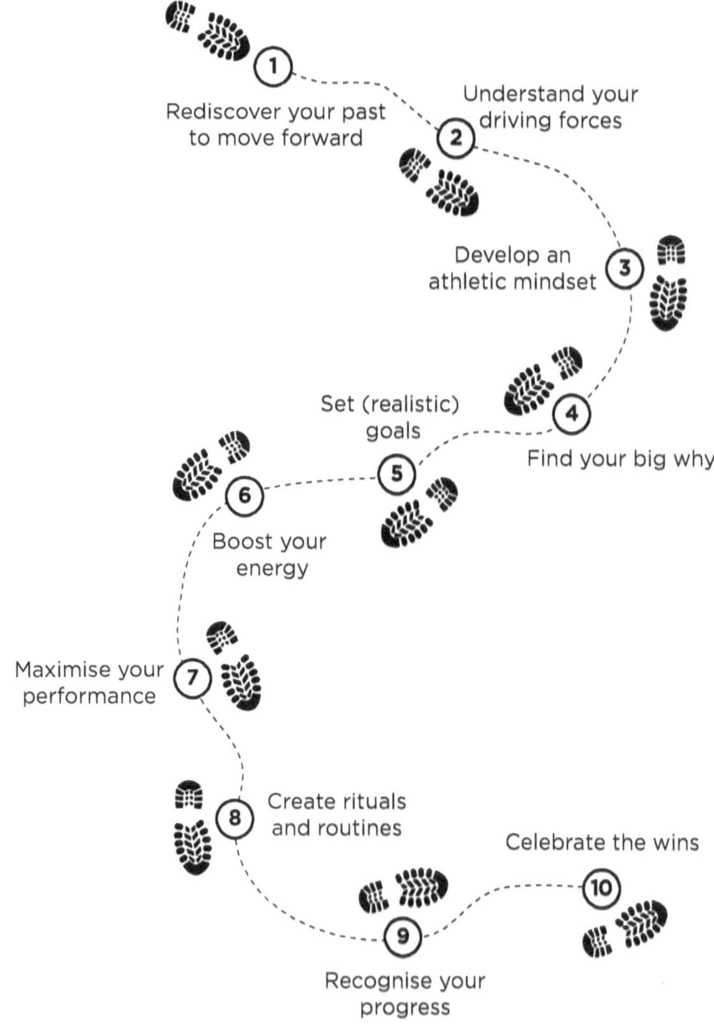

CHANGE IS NEVER EASY

Often what's easy is to follow the predictable and familiar trail, to sit back down on the couch where it's warm and comfy and make yourself a drink. Taking the ride means making a shift, crossing a gap, experiencing a period of discomfort. Decisions cause change, which means embracing the new and learning to say no. It requires putting in the effort, making a commitment, time to face the music, you have work to do. All of this involves developing the mindset and rituals that will carry you through. There are times we step into the unknown, feel the fear and do it anyway. It begins with saying yes. Just like taking a deep breath as the roller-coaster turns towards the sky.

We all know it's easy to talk ourselves out of getting on the ride in the first place. We're busy, other things are more urgent, life seems to creep up on us. We just seem to become buried under a pile of 'I can't' and 'I used to's' or – even better – 'I'm too old'. Beaten down by the past. This stops us in our tracks and keeps us where we are, not where we want to be.

Life doesn't come with a guarantee or a warranty. There comes a point we have to make a decision on what we feel inside. Not deciding is a choice in itself. Experience tells us that change is never easy, and even scary. What if it is the wrong choice and it doesn't work out?

The journey you are about to undertake will certainly be a little scary. It will have dips and dives, go fast and slow, but if you are willing to stay on the path you will rediscover your Athlete Within, and that will unleash an amazing sense of possibility for you in everything you do.

You then have the choice to stay on the ride or get off. My job is to guide you, encourage you and help you finish the ride.

SLOW AND STEADY

Wherever this book may take you, the goal is to experience a change, small or big, that impacts the rest of your life, something that truly lasts and becomes part of who you are. So for the time being, please consider where you are and keep the word 'longevity' in mind. Maybe even the word 'sustainable'. If you haven't run, skipped or jumped for a very long time, chances are you'll have to take this slow and steady. There will be no entering marathons in two months, signing up to climb Mount Everest with your friends or even joining the local touch rugby club until you have sought proper advice.

Just as this book has 10 steps, you too will need to take one step at a time in getting back in the saddle. Rediscovering your Athlete Within is not a competition, nor is it about doing it in a certain amount of time. It is about you discovering an aspect of you, maybe an old part of you, and bringing it back to life.

PART I

WHERE
YOU
ARE
NOW

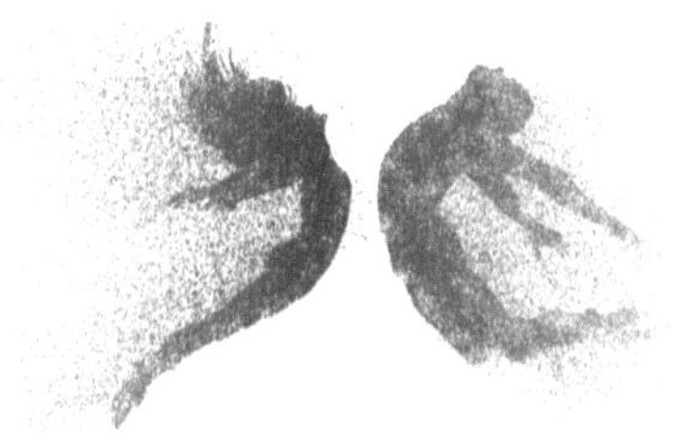

FIND A BIGGER PURPOSE

MEET JANE

And in bursts Jane.

I don't think Jane actually opened the door when she entered our clinic, she just seemed to arrive. Filled with such excitement, she unashamedly unleashed at the top of her lungs:

'I did it – I finished the walk!'

As anyone would understand, to finish the Bloody Long Walk is a feat.

To spend a day walking the 35-kilometre scenic route, strolling along the 15 different glorious beaches, is the stuff champions like Jane are made for. A charity event, the walk begins in Palm Beach and winds its way down into Manly, making for a seriously impressive challenge. Did I also mention climbing the gruelling steep headlands, dealing with onshore headwinds and the direct winter sun glaring down? But the real win for our Jane wasn't just what you see on the outside. There was also the inside job of who Jane had become before she had even shown up that day.

Eighteen months before, when I first met Jane, she was struggling to get out of bed every morning and walk the five steps to her kitchen to just greet the day. A simple netball injury years before – coming off second best from a ball challenge caused her to land heavily on her hip – resulted in a painful limp for two days. Years later, she was involved in a collision, without too much damage to her light blue '69 VW Beetle, but she reaggravated her old hip injury when she jumped heavily on the brakes. Then her house of cards came falling down. An ongoing and now degenerated hip spun into a spinal disc injury, which meant living with some serious pain more often than she could remember.

But there's more to her story.

Having it all ... ?

Jane had been left devastated when her husband of 19 years had walked out on their marriage for no particular reason except his secretary seemed like the better option. Deep down she knew it was coming – she hadn't been herself for some time. With the kids getting older and rarely at home, scoring that incredible promotion at work was now chewing up more hours than she would care to admit. They were now simply ships passing in the night. Homelife had become routine. The weekends were like small escapes for a quick breather, just enough for her to wrap up each week at a time, only to prepare for the next.

Looking back, Jane seemed to have it all: the first one in her family to graduate from university, getting snapped up by one of the top firms in her industry, it was all a dream where the pieces were just fitting into place. Then she fell in love, married, and relished a six-week honeymoon spent travelling around Europe, soaking up culture, touring endless castles and of course eating way too much food.

All too soon life took its natural course with the arrival of three beautiful children. Jane's house became a home filled with the sound of little feet. It felt like life just couldn't be better.

But the years went by and things just seemed to creep up. Money became tight, there were credit cards due, mortgage payments to make. The kids being old enough for school meant Jane re-entered the workforce. A previous law partner happy to see her return, knowing her high work ethic, snapped her up, and soon 2.5 days turned into three and occasionally four. They seemed to be getting ahead, paying off the car, taking bigger holidays, moving in the right direction. Yet the schedule was full, constantly driving kids to various dance activities, soccer training, and then Saturday was sport.

When was there time left for her?

She knew she should be taking better care of herself and for periods she did, meeting friends and going for walks, joining the gym, but none of it ever really stuck. She was stopping and starting again, always with the latest first-world family or work crisis to deal with. But she was mum, the superwoman, the one who would listen, would understand, got everyone where they needed to be on time – the glue that kept the family together.

Implosion

Wide awake at 4 o'clock one morning, her mind racing at a 100 miles per hour, frustrated about the case she was involved in at work, nothing seemed to be going her way. Rolling over for the umpteenth time, her mind wondered at her own life and how she had ended up at this point. She thought to herself, *is this how it is meant to be?*

She was now nearing another birthday – this one would tip her into the 50s club. All she could think about was how old she felt, how embarrassed she was at being so out of shape and feeling so unhappy about herself. She stopped to think back to her younger self, how she used to love to run through the bush and down along the water's edge in the evenings, never with a time in mind or breaking a record but just finding her own space. This was her element, her sense of freedom away from all the challenges of the world.

Deep down she knew she had to get herself moving again. She had to think more long term, and realised as much as she liked to get things done quickly, this would require time. Jane slept in a little longer than usual the next morning; she was tired, only getting up to go to the toilet. It was then she was struck by a lightning bolt of back pain which left her on the floor. That was the real sign that tipped the scale. Jane realised she had reached a critical point – she *had* to do something different.

That was when I first met Jane.

Overwhelmed and exhausted, she felt like she had lost her grip on life. Sitting down with Jane was touching; on the surface she held strength and determination, yet her personal story was moving. So many battles and so much emotion. Helping Jane also meant her finding her own truth, who she was meant to be.

We got to work.

Jane looked back and saw her life as a series of events, a series of moments, each being part of a bigger picture, each chapter connecting to form her own life story. She wondered what she would say to her younger self, or what her younger self would say to her today.

About this time, on one of her lunchtime walks, a friend mentioned she was forming a group for a charity walk. Jane called for a special appointment in our clinic – she felt she had come so far, it was time to discuss her future and what was possible. She floated the idea of being part of this walking team, part of something with a greater meaning and purpose. We brainstormed her gap. At this point she was successfully walking every day and was now able to run her Saturday morning 5-kilometre park run. But 35 kilometres in one day meant her gap was a … leap.

And so began our preparation and her journey, building a process, designing a framework, starting at her base camp. This way she could tick off each step, see her own progress and what was around the corner. In the background, Jane had cut back some of her work hours to help with the team preparation – this project was something bigger than just her. There was a feeling deep inside. A bigger purpose. She had found her reason to do it and she didn't stop.

'I did it – I finished the walk!' I'd had no doubts she would. Because I believed she could and so did she. More than that: Jane found and became her Athlete Within.

*

We all recognise Jane's story, because as much as we try, life doesn't always go to plan. There is conflict, mistakes and pain where we can either get stuck or we can use it to grow to become our own greatness. Jane was living life, ticking all the boxes, juggling all the balls and doing what she thought was right. Yet things didn't turn out as she expected. She had to stop, regroup and make decisions along the way. It is in these moments she created a different version of herself, something that held a greater meaning.

It is this story and many others that help us recognise our own Athlete Within.

We each have our own unique life story, our library of experiences and our list of dreams to choose from. That challenges us about whether we are living our best life. Whether it is time for a new chapter.

Maybe you are Jane and her story is very familiar.

Where do you find yourself now?

Are you ready to rediscover your Athlete Within?

Notes

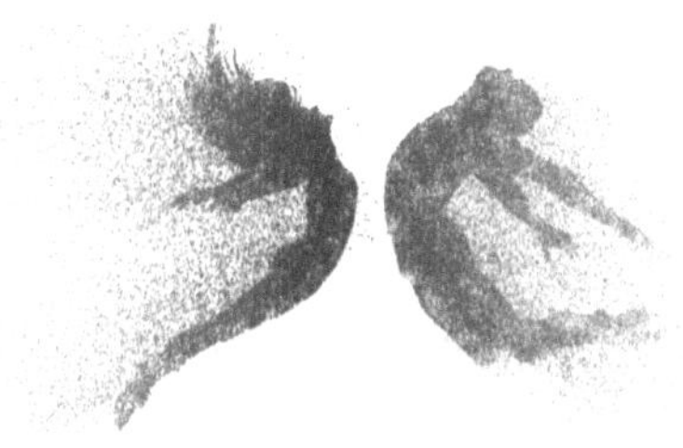

THE BEGINNING OF BEING AN ATHLETE

DO YOU REMEMBER WHEN ... ?

It's the middle of the school holidays, the peak of winter. The wind has a certain chill to it that tastes of snow and this year we chose the beach as our holiday destination. Filled with ideas of building sandcastles, walks up to the lighthouse and BBQs for dinner. How wrong did we get that ...

Kids just change the plans; they see the world in a totally different way. On this occasion they clearly did not read the brochure. Beach means surf, surf means splashing in the water. Of course we didn't pack the swimmers – we got this, the undies will be just fine. In the end you talk them out of the ocean, the final straw being their little lips turning blue, hiding chattering teeth. It's back to the bungalow. Of course, the bungalow is decked out with a pool and a water park. Open the gate, it just starts all over again. Remember that age when the fun outweighs the cold?

Remember when you were a kid, what you got up to? It was crazy. It was fun. It was the stuff dreams are made of. Childhood was where all your hopes and ambitions about life began. The rules didn't apply. Responsibilities weren't law. Getting kicked outside for making too much noise. You were unstoppable. When going on a car trip was boring and sitting still and being quiet required something called patience. Yawn. Life was full, it was fun to play, where a park only needed a swing for entertainment.

In these moments you were planting the seeds of your Athlete Within. The construction of concepts and definitions. Of memories tied up in games, joining in, being active. Where learning – and sometimes making – the rules happened while you played the game. Where the fun was being part of the gang. We all shared winning, we all got a turn. Now you are older, you look around and ask, 'Where do they get all that energy? When do they ever stop?'

But the real question is, when did *you* stop?

Of course we all have our moments of greatness, not all of them on the sports field. There are your 'firsts': your first bike, your first three-legged race, your first tap shoes or trampoline if you're lucky.

Or great memories of being a kid – out on your bike for hours, kicking a ball with your mates, cartwheels at lunch down at the oval. It was all tied up with being active, laughing and having the time of our life. These moments we often shared with family and friends, where no one really kept score, it wasn't about the win, competing or doing a PB. The rules were letting loose, having fun, classic catches, enjoying each other's company, soaking up the moments.

Let's dive a little further. Who was your greatest athletic hero growing up? Can you pick just one? I grew up with images of Grant Kenny jumping through the waves, the Nutri-Grain commercials – Iron Man food. I remember my grandfather always had sport on somewhere, even if it was just the radio out in the garden, prompting another game of backyard cricket with the neighbours.

Back to today – everything is moving so fast, working to deadlines, running to be on time, a quick break for lunch. Never stopping to recognise our own wins. We are so caught up juggling balls, exhausted with overflowing to-do lists. We are hard on ourselves, noticing every time we drop the ball, forget something or turn up late. All of this creeps up on us with time, until we lose belief in ourselves, in our own ability. The next time someone pulls out a ball and says let's play, you are reluctant, feeling like you will miss and make a fool out of yourself. You've already outplayed yourself in your head.

Remembering is a chance to go back and dig up those good times. Memories are more than tiny stories of our past, they are your history, your emotional library, the recipes that made you who you are today. Looking back is an opportunity to relive the magic – remember the moments that made you laugh and smile – and reconnect. Seeing how your decisions shaped the person you are. It strengthens your understanding of yourself.

Remembering is connecting with your story, decide if it needs to be updated with a new perspective.

THE GAP

'When a man says he has exhausted life, one always knows life has exhausted him.'

Oscar Wilde

Good decision-making is a key characteristic of an athlete.

But what is it that holds us back when making decisions? What makes us want to stick our head in the sand or continue travelling the known path? Often there is a change we desire, a promise we dream of. What stands in the way is a gap we need to cross, filled with 'unknowns' and 'not nows'. The thing is, you have made it across gaps in the past, many times.

Crossing the gap begins with an internal agreement about why you want to cross this gap, getting yourself out of the way and taking the first step. Decisions don't come with a guarantee. As we walk the path between chaos and order, it is our wisdom that guides us. The context is more than just the existing conditions, it is our previous experiences and concerns, as well as our future expectations. It is a feeling we hold on to that keeps us stuck to the old path:

- It's hard.
- I'm tired.
- I'm too old now.
- I'll start tomorrow.
- I have the kids to deal with.
- I haven't got the money.
- What if it doesn't work?
- I need to wash the car.
- My work is full-on at the moment.
- My partner tries to understand.
- I need to do this other thing first.
- You don't understand the pressures I'm under.
- I can't remember the last time I bounced out of bed with energy.
- Maybe I am just happy the way I am.
- I have tried it so many times before.
- I'm just not ready yet.
- My doctor says I'm okay.
- I don't feel heard.
- I'm worried.

What causes us to make decisions? To make serious changes in our life? To start something new?

Change is never easy. If it was easy, it wouldn't really be a change. Trying something new requires making a decision, a process of assessment followed by real commitment. Often we cling to a story, comfortable just the way things are. To change would be to open up a door, take a risk, expose ourselves, step into vulnerability – the consequence being growth. Comfortable just means the world is meeting our expectations. We have a sense of control but life holds little surprise. Why do we cling on? Because our stories give us meaning in the moment and a predictable identity. But stories can also be an insight into our own narrative. To shift is to step into the unknown and create growth.

'Life is either a daring adventure or nothing at all.'

Hellen Keller

Many of the decisions we make satisfy a short-term need. It's New Year's Eve, you make a list of resolutions, you finally decide the next day you will join the gym. You start living the dream and loving the honeymoon period. Then things start to happen – the tests. You stay back late at work, you didn't bring your runners, and gently the five times a week falls back to three times a week. But you're okay with this. It's all part of the plan, and three times a week is what they recommend, right? By April, the wheels have fallen off. You still make it twice a week … mostly. But who are we kidding? The plan really needs a bigger engine if it's going to last the distance.

THE BIGGER ENGINE

Rediscovering your Athlete Within is a process that starts with your story. You know you, the ups and downs, the pitfalls and mountain tops. Unless you are dedicated and you make a real commitment, your plan is not going to last the test of time. The reality is, sustainability and longevity come down to your amount of buy-in in the first place. I love to ask new clients if they have that exercise bike or treadmill which has morphed into a clothes horse.

How do you go about making decisions? Is it a strong character trait in you that you are proud of? I'm talking about creating clarity, redefining the question so it is clear, understanding the context and circumstances, then making a decision you can hang your hat on. Good decision-making is about working with failure. The ultimate aim is understanding that failure is a key learning process for the human species.

Why you do what you do

If you're not sure what your bigger engine is, start by thinking about these questions:

- What are your favourite hobbies?
- When was the last time you really laughed out loud?
- What is your favourite movie?
- What music do you listen to?
- What is your favourite restaurant?
- Who are the top three people you love to spend time with?
- Who would you most like to have dinner with?
- What is the last book you read?
- What two things matter the most to you?
- How would your partner or a close friend describe you?
- Write a list of your best seven qualities – why do people love being around you?
- What are your five top beliefs?
- What are three qualities you want to practise more of?
- What are seven things you want to do more of?

- Is there enough adventure and risk in your life?
- Is your life organised and structured?
- Do you arrive on time?
- Do you finish things?

The whole purpose of 'rediscovering' you is to find out what resonates. What do you really want?

Notes

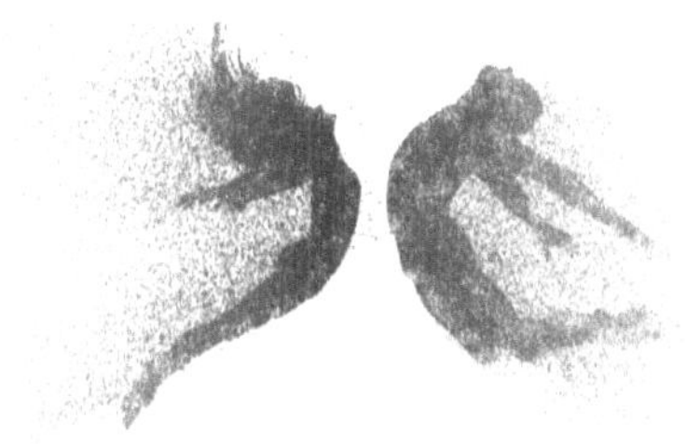

YOU DON'T HAVE TO
ACT YOUR AGE

MOVING FROM THE AM TO THE PM OF YOUR LIFE

Bronnie Ware, a palliative nurse, wrote the incredible book *The Top Five Regrets of the Dying*. In it she discusses the top five lessons she has taken from the dying:

- find more courage
- spend less time at work
- express your true self
- stay in touch
- let yourself be happier.

How often do we take time to contemplate life? The reality is our lives are constantly changing, winding and weaving, tending to follow a general script, yet we all still trail off into our own versions. The previous section prompted you to think about the decisions shaping our lives, and now we are turning our attention to the PM years. Stopping to see where we are makes sense, yet how often do we actually take the time? We joke about the midlife crisis and carrying regrets – this is almost an accepted part of the process – only to realise we've lived on autopilot and strayed from our own identity, what makes us who we are. It is time to turn your attention to the bigger questions in life.

Like a rite of passage of a child becoming an adult member of the tribe, the shift from the 40s and 50s into the PM years should celebrate fresh new hope. From the morning to the afternoon of our life. There was a time when growing older was respected. You were treated gratefully for your knowledge, experience and advice, and referred to as an 'elder'. The old ways are being left behind in our fast, technologically driven lifestyles.*

There is a shift in values that changes our perspective on life, affecting our expectations. I caught one of my friends telling his teenager he is 'too old to do that anymore'. Are you? Or are you just letting it slip away?

In our 20s and 30s we tend to look more to the outside, towards the physical stuff. It's all about time, achievement, fulfilling expectations. We put our heads down and follow predestined pathways without too many questions, following a career path, starting a family, hopefully buying a house and enjoying some holidays. With age, these adventures of youth tend to fade, the roads narrow, become more dirt tracks, not tending to make sense like they once did. Those middle years become a turning point, towards a more internal and deeper understanding of life. We start to ask the bigger questions. As you hit the afternoon of life, the rules that governed the morning don't apply. Many of us lose sight of the bigger picture.

We might be looking for big, instant changes: a new, maybe younger, partner. We drop everything and travel or buy a motorbike. Some make a gentler transition, follow the same career path well into

---

* This is eloquently put by Professor Wayne Dyer in his book *The Shift: Taking Your Life from Ambition to Meaning.*

their 70s, only to ask the big questions lying on their deathbed. As Talking Heads put it, 'Well, how did I get here?'

For many of us there is a jolt of awakening that lands on our doorstep; a misadventure, a death, financial chaos, a divorce or serious illness. In a sense, a point where the decision is thrust upon us. This is a shift from the external to the more internal, more spiritual. A time when you may slow down, shift into a different gear, and your thoughts turn more to understanding, meaning and your own life.

Rediscovering your Athlete Within is about hitting the middle parts of your life with new energy and new reasoning and finding purpose. An opportunity to take a breath, reach out and navigate the next chapter forward.

I remember a conversation with my grandmother when she was 95 years old, laughing about the fact it gets easier to say 'no' the older we get. After living through World Wars and depressions, life goes on, and she told me it was our job to grow with it. Saying no means you become clearer about what is important, and with it you grow a thicker skin.

When was the last time you thought about what life looks like in your PM years? What adjustments should you be making in the now? Think back to a time when you had a conversation with an elder; what was said, what did you learn? Why did that moment impact you? Are you on track towards a life well lived?

*

Our ancestors were remarkable, mastering how to be upright, figuring out how to think better, think ahead, use and develop tools, build a tribe and develop speech and then language. They became runners, they developed endurance, they learnt how to acquire food diversity through growing skills in hunting and foraging, and learnt the art of sharing, probably one of the biggest keys to our survival. They lived through famines, plagues, predators and everything else Mother Earth could throw at them, yet still they evolved. You are the latest model of this incredible line of success stories. What is your story going to be?

At birth you were handed a Version 3.0 model that came out of the factory of Mother Nature. It included an operating system with the most advanced features and upgrades already installed. Of course, evolution has stress-tested its capabilities and made required adaptions to meet environmental demands and conditions. We turned tools into technology, creative became innovative, our nomadic past driving forward through the agricultural era, the industrial era, the information era to today's era of technology. We stand on the shoulders of millions of years of evolution.

So if we are living our best life ever … why doesn't it feel like it?

It's all about reframing your understanding of what ageing is, injecting your version of an athlete to take advantage of the opportunities that lie ahead. So, what is biologically possible? Our bodies, given the right environment and way of life, have the potential to live to 120 years, or even 150 years. We have become smarter, more capable, more adaptable, but not necessarily stronger or faster. We live longer with more leisure and pleasure, but not necessarily better.

The stats are in your favour. If you were born in the 1940s like my mum, your life expectancy is around 63 years. Today this sits in the mid-80s. One in three Aussie kids will become centenarians. A 10 year old has a 50% chance of living to a 104 years. No surprise the centenarians are the fastest growing segment in today's population; they are overtaking the planet. America has 800,000 centenarians, Japan is a close second with 500,000. What do you have to do to live 100 birthdays? Just grow old, right? The bottom line: the older you get, the greater the chance you will get even older.

THE CRITICAL WINDOW

But stop … there is a bigger conversation to be had: assuming you're well on your way to 100, how will you actually live out those PM years?

It's easy to plan the next three months, talk through ideas for the next five years, but seldom do we plan 12 years ahead or more.

The 50s club is a turning point. Your body shifts gears. Statistically it's where life catches up and you meet challenges in the form of illness and disease. Your body can also experience transitions, such as menopause, all of which slow you down. The science shows that how you spend your 40s and 50s will largely determine the quality of your PM years. It is a critical window.

What does that mean for you? Now is the time you want to rediscover your Athlete Within.

Let's wake you up for a moment. Do you know what you are bound to deal with when you hit 50? The list is long. Coronary heart disease is the leading cause of death up to 64. If your cholesterol and blood pressure are high, you have 10 times greater risk of a heart attack. Starting at 65 years of age, your risk of Alzheimer's disease doubles every five years. If you are over the age of 60 you are 90% likely to be carrying around a chronic condition, and if you are 70 then you are 80% likely to be walking around with at least two chronic conditions.

Just getting you thinking about your future is key. Thinking about your own impact on how you live, earlier, sets a new direction and way of life.

Ageing is a normal part of any biological cycle whether it be degeneration, deterioration or erosion. At the end of the day it is the inability of a cell to accurately replicate itself. Think of it like this: every time you take a photocopy, the image looks the same, but with each copy it loses a sharpness, a focus, some definition of detail.

In research, scientists take this seriously, studying 'pathological ageing', the processes that speed up ageing. The biggest player? Lifestyle. Exercise, activity level, behaviour, all the way through to the quality of our sleep and circadian cycles. Scientists look at balancing biochemistry, energy expenditure equations, cleaning out toxic rubbish and making repairs. But also the significance of keeping within our natural habitual rhythms, both in our internal world as well as our external environment. We are entering an era where the way we live is the greatest impact on longevity and quality of life. An era where age is not just a number – your chronological age – but reflects the quality of life you are living – your biological age.

But wait, there's more. The good news is coming. What kind of lifestyle is conducive to a long and healthy life? There is Blue Zone thinking where researchers are investigating specific locations where large pockets of centenarians live to study their lifestyle and habits. In 1981, 18,000 residents in a retirement village once referred to as 'Leisure World' in – where else – California took a detailed survey examining many factors about the way they lived. Today this group of people over 90 are referred to as the 'Older Oldies', forming the basis of a string of research into what longevity looks like. One of these researchers is Dr Claudia Kawas, who led the study of the Laguna Woods residents. Her findings make so much sense to me, because they align with the Athlete Within:

- Exercising at least 15 minutes a day affected longevity in the participants. Those who exercised moderately for 45 minutes or longer per day lived longer.

- People who drank moderate amounts of alcohol or coffee (one serve a day each) lived longer than those who didn't.

- Residents were socially active: they read, played bridge and other games, plus enjoyed a little romance on the side.

As you drop some of the baggage of the AM years, embrace saying no, living more in line with your own truth, it also means finding your own athletic self. Living your best life means taking care of your body as if it is your most valued treasure. Let's face it, if you haven't got your health, it's hard to enjoy an incredible life.

Are you thinking about how you're living right now and how your lifestyle could impact your PM years? We all want to say *yes* but do we stop to think about what that might actually look like? This is your time for action. This is your critical window.

THESE ARE YOUR GOLDEN YEARS

In 2004 on a trip to Prague, I encountered one of those moments we have all experienced: you meet someone who defies the laws of gravity and time.

Jiří Čumpelík was a retired professional ballet dancer, now a leading authority in functional movement. In 2004, I was part of a group of Australians who found ourselves on a wooden floor, attempting to follow his direction and emulate how a 'baby' learns to roll. It was horrible. Our Aussie ears found it difficult to understand his thick accent, so he promptly popped on the floor and demonstrated the exercises himself with grace and agility. Probably half his age, we struggled to follow, let alone keep up. It then became a game about guessing how old this guy was. He looked old, but the way he could use his body left us speechless. It's not like he didn't age, he just didn't act his age.

A lot of us grow up with preconceptions about what it means to get old. As we reach old, we just begin to act out these stories: 'you start, I'll catch up'. I think maybe it has more to do with having a reason to live life and more so the PM of our life.

So if age is more than just a number, what do your golden years look like? If I asked you to describe what 82 years old looks like, who would you start to picture?

Notes

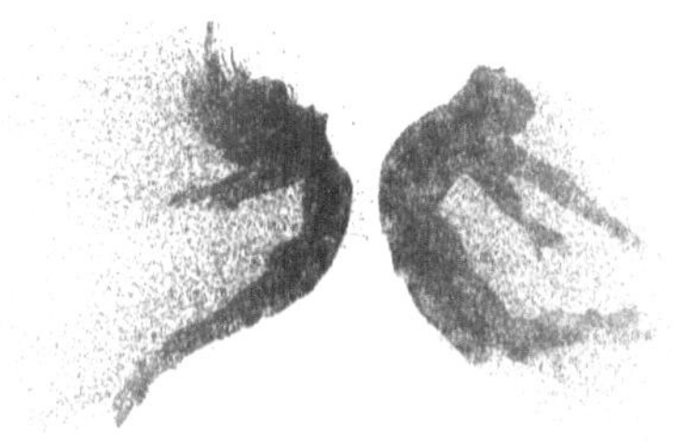

OPEN THE DOOR TO POSSIBILITY

YOUR WISHLIST

We seem to keep a dream wishlist in our head that only ever remains that, a dream, something far ahead in the distance. What if we created our wishlist and started ticking it off today? We all walk around with these ideas floating in our head of 'one day' that would be really great. But when does that one day ever come?

We are here, now. So what do you desire? What are your dreams? What lies on the realms of possibility, what could be? What if you were done waiting and every day for the next week you woke up with a clean page and wrote 20 things down. Where would you go? What would you do? What is the craziest thing? What is the most fun thing?

What would just make you laugh? What would be a moment you would want to slow down for and cherish?

This is the magic we all want. What could you be proud of? Who do you want to be? It's time to start writing your ultimate wishlist without fear, without worry about the nitty gritty. Just step into the moment and be free. And if you find it hard to start your list, think back to what you wanted to become or do when you were a kid. What were some of your wishes then?

Dream and then dream some more. You're made for a life well lived. To rediscover your Athlete Within means taking the best of who you are and designing the life of (you guessed it) your dreams.

EMBRACING UNCERTAINTY

There is something about heights. Many years ago, I skied in beautiful Jackson Hole. High up, by myself on a sky lift, I was doing a last run before calling it quits. My ride came to a grinding halt, leaving me swinging way up in the air. Long minutes passed. Then my mind woke up. With the light fading, I realised there was no one on the seats in front of me, or behind. Slowly panic set in. Was I going to be stuck here all night?

Fast forward 15 years, I am away with an incredible group of friends, out for an early morning adventure. Driving through the dark in the back country above beautiful Florence, we come to a stop in the middle of a random field. Hot-air balloons are waiting for us on the cold morning grass. Instantly I am taken back to Jackson Hole.

No, I'm not going up in a hot-air balloon. *You don't understand, I have history.* My head takes over and my mind quickly goes into a panic. Suddenly everything is like a tunnel. I approach the organiser, who is surprised by my strong reaction. The pressure is only mine and I have a choice. I realise my ripple effect on others, as they start swallowing hard, unsure about their own feelings of going up.

A close friend holds my hand tight and makes a pact. 'I will stay with you, we've got this … but the choice is yours.' There is a moment when her eyes hold mine, in that early morning light, still crystal bright in my memory. I breathe out, move my body out of rigidity and answer, 'Let's do this'.

Every process comes with its own adventures. We are all familiar with the feeling of stepping out into the storm. It is time to work, time to stretch. We relinquish control, brace for what we sense is coming, and increase the effort to make it through. We all sense there is still more inside. Our brain is a protector. It has been a survival machine for eons. It's just keeping us safe. But is safe what life is about? Remember that saying, a ship is safe in the harbour, but is that what it was built for?

You realise it's your time, where embracing uncertainty requires a deeper trust. You do it because something inside of you speaks to you. It is a feeling, call it a truth. If we put out a challenge, the universe responds by checking in to see if we are serious. Throwing a little problem here, an obstacle there. It is all part of the process. Rising through this shows you are willing to step up to the line and take your place.

Everything in your life leads up to this point.

Just like taking the roller-coaster ride.

There comes a point where the analysis is done.

Your heart says yes.

It's your turn.

Step up onto the ride.

On your marks.

Set.

Go.

Notes

PART II

—

THE
ATHLETE
WITHIN
FRAMEWORK

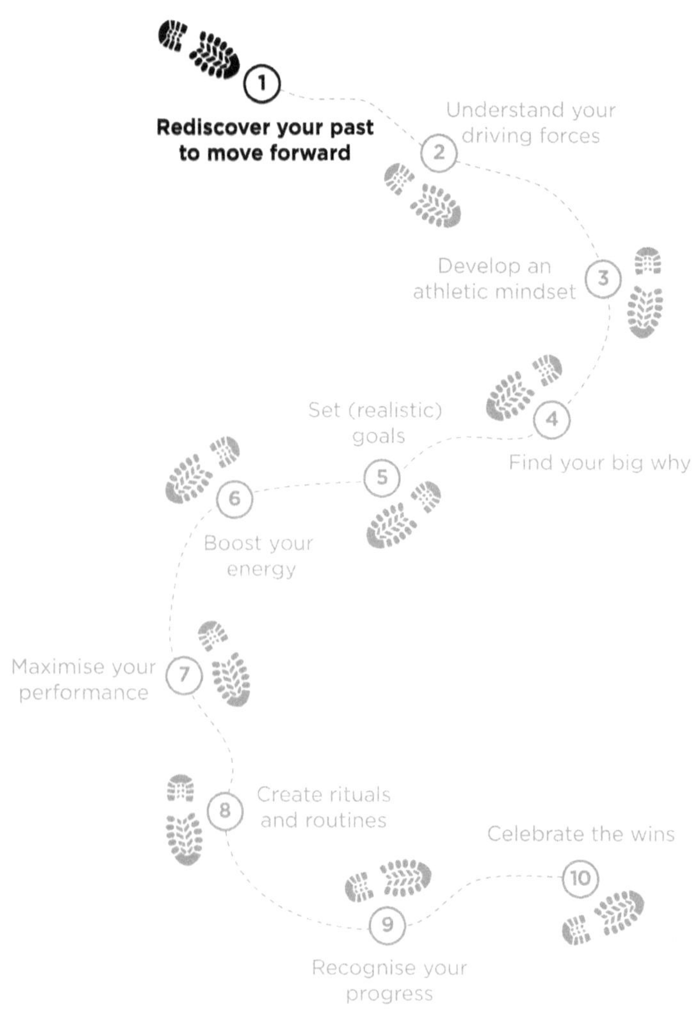

1
Rediscover your past to move forward
Understand your driving forces
2
Develop an athletic mindset
3
Find your big why
4
Set (realistic) goals
5
Boost your energy
6
Maximise your performance
7
Create rituals and routines
8
Recognise your progress
9
Celebrate the wins
10

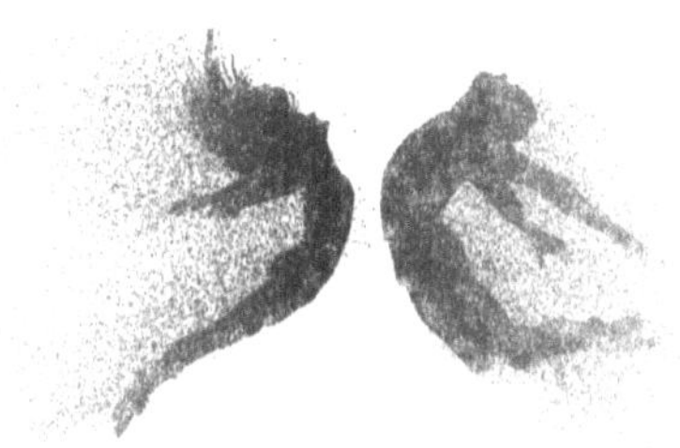

STEP 1:
REDISCOVER YOUR PAST
TO MOVE FORWARD

WHO IS YOUR ATHLETE WITHIN?

John was an executive banker who came to our clinic complaining his spine clicked a little. Each time he stood up there would be a chorus of clicks like someone running a hammer along a xylophone. Of course he knew it wasn't right, but there was never any pain. It was his wife that scheduled the appointment and sent him in.

When John was growing up he played rugby. He loved it. His school had multiple teams, from A-grade down to F-grade. John was much smaller compared to the other boys so he was relegated to the F team, which he and his friends affectionately named the 'failures'. John had no chance of climbing up the grades. He didn't shoot up in height and size until much later in his teens; he was almost 16 years old and too late for a rugby career. You can almost imagine the moment when John lost his athletic confidence.

John had followed the well-trodden path, working hard climbing the career ladder. Life was more about sitting, and then when he arrived home, his main hobby was reading, requiring more sitting. The writing was on the wall. There had been periods of starting at the gym or walking outdoors, but – John being relatively famous – these episodes were usually interrupted with media interactions he would rather avoid. Over the years his body had slowly slumped down the slippery slope of deconditioning. What was once a picture of physical strength in his 20s had morphed into a much less robust version of a man, carrying a little extra something around the waist. The urgency of his work had kept him occupied, he married a little later in life, and his beautiful son was now growing up.

Walking out of his first appointment, he was thinking about his own mortality and the road he was currently travelling. It was over the weekend, when he saw his wife and son outside by the pool, that he thought he would head out to join them. Perhaps clean up a few of those leaves that had floated down onto the surface. Picking up the long handle of the pool cleaner, he collected the leaves and then settled into his pool lounge with a good book. The next morning he struggled to get out of bed; he now had pain, to the entertainment of his 13-year-old son and concern of his wife. The mental image he had of his body didn't match his reality, his athletic self. His true self was starting to speak up, loudly.

Over the weeks, John had been following his program, building his Athlete Within with floor exercises to re-train his spine. He was developing more strength and functionality in his frame, and his confidence was growing. As he started to spend more time out at the pool, sweeping the leaves from the surface of the water, he was having more conversations with his son. More chit chat, how his son's day had turned out, what exams were coming up. These conversations grew into the pressures his son was feeling, assignments piling up, trying to get along with difficult kids at school. John got on well with his son, yet now he realised his son needed him more. His son was changing, growing up, thinking about the bigger questions in life that didn't come up over the dinner table.

During one appointment in the clinic, a conversation led him to buy two baseball gloves, and he started playing catch with his son and spending more time with him in the late afternoon sun. Soon the two of them, messing around, ended up wrestling on the ground. Their relationship grew, it evolved, it was like they were reuniting on a deeper level, sharing a lot more about each other. John made some big realisations. It was like he rediscovered his own Athlete Within, just at the time his son needed him the most.

There are a million ways to be your own athlete; you just need to rediscover yours. I believe inside every one of us is an athlete, an active little kid that has already spent hours perfecting their own skills and knows how to play their own game.

Yet we fell into the trap. We just forgot.

THE SECRET IS IN YOUR PAST

'Those who fail to learn from history are doomed to repeat it.'

Sir Winston Churchill

When was the last time you sat down and flicked through your old photo albums, remembering all the stories of how it was growing up? Our memories can let emotions bubble up to the surface so we connect to something we truly cherish, but they can also show us mistakes we learned from. Remembering is a process of walking back into the matrix and connecting, searching and following rabbit holes, and then sitting back and being amazed to see what pops up. Our past holds a lot of clues about who we are, some of them more significant than others, some where we can feel it in our gut. It is these points that have greater meaning and possible connection to a deeper root inside us. These are the memories you want to capture, the light bulb moments that flash more brightly and bring out tears of laughter or sadness.

People sometimes tell me they don't know what they want to do or they don't know what they are good at. This is why going back into your past is important and is also so much fun – not just remembering the things you used to get up to but also the hours and hours of your childhood spent being active and busy, where time stopped and everything was an adventure. You were on. These clues can lead you back to understanding what you really loved doing, your tendencies and your passions. All of this is unlocking your Athlete Within.

Become an observer

As you go back into your past, stay in a position of being the observer. Try not to go back into the experience but see it from a distance. We are looking for the light bulb moments that shaped you, the things you developed a passion for, what you found easy and related to.

By going back in time you can see where your passions came to life and how, what you were excited about and what you woke up in the morning dreaming about.

Hindsight is *knowing what you know now, what would you tell yourself back then?* Life gives us experience and a way to interpret ourselves; this is wisdom, the ability to see something as separate as well as in context, to understand its relevance, its significance, and to see how it played out.

Ask your family or friends for stories about the things you used to get up to and they will share not just the funny but the unique: what made you special, what you were good at, what you did that was just *you*.

Exercise

Hindsight is a great teacher. With it you can see things in context, make links, understand associations and how patterns and habits emerged. As you think back to your past, give yourself the gift of time to uncover moments, clues that can help you rediscover your little athlete.

Can you see how these clues can help you determine your Athlete Within of today?

I remember my father mowing our back lawn, the smell of cut grass, being told not to go too close to the Jasmine bush because of the bees, then hiding behind the bush with my mum finding me. My little athlete was running, hiding, digging in the garden, laughing as I was picked up and swung around.

I remember preschool, going to a big hall with other kids. There was this red tricycle I used to love riding around and around. Our street had a cul-de-sac where we would join the other kids and kick a ball at the park at the top of the hill. There were swings, a red phone box and lots of bush to run in and play soldiers. There was a family holiday at the beach. There were birthday parties, blowing out candles. I remember making kites out of old newspaper and bamboo with my best friend Paul, and heading up to the park to fly them.

I remember starting high school, entering cross-country for my age group then moving into the open adult category later, and how they were all slow running up the hill, exhausted as I overtook them. I remember when I stopped playing cricket and followed my best friend Jason into baseball. Such a new sport, the rules so different, so many innings, but we seemed to get to play every position. The novelty of this new game drew me in. They thought I was a natural, but at home I practised for hours throwing a ball against the front brick wall of the house.

I listen to my wife's stories as she remembers her little athlete growing up in Switzerland. She remembers skiing before she could even ride a bike. Winter was her wonderland as she zipped down the hills, soaking up the freedom. She tells me of the first time she went skiing. Her dad gave her a beanie, mitts, goggles and an old pair of skis. He then helped her on the lift and told her to wait at the top so he could teach her the fundamentals: she had to learn to stop first before even attempting to go. Of course, once at the top, she didn't wait. She wanted to do it all by herself, confident in her own (non-existent) abilities. And down the hill she went.

It is important to stop and remember your story because dotted along your timeline are lessons and moments that define who you are right now and what your Athlete Within is. Your story shows you how your life evolves and how patterns have formed, and helps you recognise the way you make sense of the world.

What is your story? What do you tell the kids? What do you brag about at a BBQ, or smile about when it comes up at a family lunch? We hold the secrets and fabrics of our athletes in the past. The likes, the dreams, the hopes, the successes, the lessons. It's all there. It's time to go back to your story.

Exercise

What is one of your favourite memories as a little athlete?

What did you do?

What did you feel?

How would you describe it to someone?

How does it make you feel today?

THE THREE SPHERES OF YOUR ATHLETIC PROFILE

It's time to explore the elements that make up your athletic profile. I see these as three spheres that hold your physical, cognitive and emotional essence.

The physical sphere

The physical aspect of your athlete can be described simply as *the way you are built*.

In the clinic, people often became frustrated with their body shapes, their abilities (or lack of) and the way they go about things. Why is it some people see something once and tend to pick it up straight away while others (the frustrated ones) need to work hard at it until they get it right?

Dr Stuart McGill brought this concept further to my attention. His approach to weightlifting begins with understanding the shape and make up of someone's frame because in our body types and genetic make-up lie our athletic inclinations. Slovenians, for example, are the best at deadlifts. They can pick up massive weights from the floor thanks to a more shallow shape of their hip joint. Yet don't ask a Scotsman to even attempt a deadlift as their body shape could see them break a bone. Their hips are deeper so they're not great for bending, however they are perfectly built for power. Don't let a kilt fool you, the Scots are true strong men, able to easily lift atlas stones, run a distance then pop them up on a plinth.

The way we are built is in some ways similar to a car. If you're a 4WD you can go offroad on rugged terrain, but if you're a sports car you just concentrate on racking up speed along a straight road. Some of us are more built like antelopes – tall, slender and fast on our feet – while others are more built for power, not as flexible in a yoga class yet great at moving furniture.

The cognitive sphere

Your cognitive sphere determines *how you take in and analyse information.*

People have different tendencies when it comes to learning; we all have our unique way of working things out. Our twins are the perfect example of this. Ryder, our ever-so-physical girl, learns by trial and error. Like the little bulldozer she is, she is driven by physicality and learns by repeating things multiple times until she reaches the result she's satisfied with. It doesn't matter to her whether she gets it right at first or not, she just keeps going until she does get it. Scarlett, our analytical princess, is more of a thinker and observes everything until she's made sense of it. She often appears slower at things, more cautious, where in actual fact she's just processing what's required before taking action. This very cognitive way of learning may not require as many attempts, yet when Scarlett reaches the point of being ready, she displays a high level of accuracy.

The emotional sphere

The last element of your athletic profile is your emotional sphere, which *determines how you feel about what's going on around you.*

We are attracted to particular games, sports or movements very much depending on our emotional disposition. Some of us are more team orientated, preferring to work in a partnership or group, playing a part towards the whole. Others are more inclined towards individual pursuits, working through a challenge single-mindedly on their own.

As you can begin to appreciate, different temperaments better suit different types of athletic endeavours. Some will like things to be fast, reactive, unpredictable and highly competitive, while others prefer slow, repetitive, strategic, low-impact activities where they can take their time to make decisions and problem solve.

*

Whichever sphere is more prominent in you, the distinction between the physical, cognitive and emotional aspects can help you better understand your characteristics and what you may find yourself better suited for. It will also help you understand the reasons behind your choices, successes and even challenges. For example, if you are constantly injuring or straining yourself, overloading the system, it may mean you need to consider more of your inherent physical characteristics and either learn to work within them or look at other options.

At the end of the day, the activity you choose to pursue needs to align with and satisfy your spheres.

Exercise

So let's think now about your physical, cognitive and emotional inclinations and start creating your athletic profile.

Which sphere do you resonate more with?

What particular element of each sphere sings to you?

Are you competitive? And if so, against yourself or someone else?

DISCOVER YOUR KEY PATTERNS

By now you are truly deep into rediscovering your past. As you look back, you are starting to get a sense for what memories come up strongly, the things you used to enjoy and why you loved them so much. You might even begin to connect some dots, see the links, and realise that there are patterns in the way you have approached your world and chosen to live your life up to now. From the vantage point of your older self you can now see where these patterns started to take shape and the direction they took.

Your key patterns demonstrate what you have a passion for, the pace and the way you like to do things, the intensity, even the level of difficulty. When you begin to see these links in your past, threads that keep coming up, you can start to explore different possibilities that fit into your three spheres, your predispositions, as well as your patterns.

Fiona Wright once told me Owen reached an age where he had to pick one thing; he loved soccer, he loved surfing and he loved dancing. He had great ability to work his body with accuracy, to create movement and position, in a way he could bring that movement to life. Through what he loved he developed skills that could be applied to many sports, and in fact he could have excelled in any one of these three. He had options. However, he had to choose: he could only dedicate time and focus to develop further and mature in one discipline or become average at all three.

He is now a well-known face on the surfing circuit, and when he's on the board he almost looks as if he's dancing with the waves. I often wonder if, in a sliding door moment, he could have become a great ballet dancer or soccer player. The foundations were there. So were the patterns.

Nowadays we have so many options. We can think of any activity we want to try and a club or a group or someone is offering it near where we live. It's amazing really. The number of people flocking to Forest in Alpine Victoria to participate in mountain biking has grown extensively in recent years, so that even the government is contributing to building more of these tracks. What is exciting is now trails are built in a way that not only attracts riders of all different levels but they have also been adapted for riders with disabilities. Every Athlete Within has a chance to shine.

Exercise

When you look back, what are the patterns you can start to see in yourself?

What were you more interested in? What did you find yourself exploring and repeating without needing to be told? What were your dreams, your hopes, your aspirations, and how far did you pursue them?

Looking at all this, can you now take it a step further and start thinking about the possibilities ahead? What could you try? What activity could align with your Athlete Within today?

MAP YOUR ATHLETIC ZONES

It's now time to pull it all together. Your athletic moments at these particular points in time will show your patterns and create your athletic zones, the areas of interest where you're in line with your Athlete Within. They don't have to be the same; in fact, chances are they will be different because you have grown and changed through the years. The athletic zones are your magic moments and they also give you an idea of what you think is possible. What you were and what you can become again. What you loved and how it made you feel.

What is one of your earliest memories of your athletic self? What where you doing? What did you enjoy most about this moment as your athletic self? What was your athletic profile? What skills did you learn or master in that moment?

Now think of a memory of your athletic self during primary school.

Another during secondary school.

How about when you were 18? Or in your 20s, 30s and 40s?

Take a moment to really reconnect to your past.

Exercise

As you look back and reflect on this list of experiences:

- How do they relate or connect together (look for the threads of your athletic self)? Was there a theme or an interest? Who were you when you were being this athletic self?

- At what age did you learn your greatest athletic lesson or experience your greatest athletic moment? What did you overcome as your Athlete Within? How did this shape the person you have become today (your identity)? How did this help you in life?

- Look for the tendencies, the interests picked up along the way. What characteristics do you recognise in your athletic self?

- Physical characteristics – did you enjoy the effort to climb a mountain or just the physicality of being your athletic self?

- Cognitive characteristics – how did you tend to learn new things, new games, new activities, new techniques? Maybe you enjoyed the strategy and putting the game into action?

- Emotional characteristics – what was it about being your athletic self that made you feel alive? How did you feel when you were having the time of your life as your athletic self?

- How would you describe your greatest athletic moment?

- As you look back over your athletic lifetime, what inspires you the most? How does thinking about this moment make you feel now? What is one detail that stands out for you?

- What did you like most about your athletic self as you were growing up?

- What one quality or story of your athletic self can you take away and share with your loved ones?

Notes

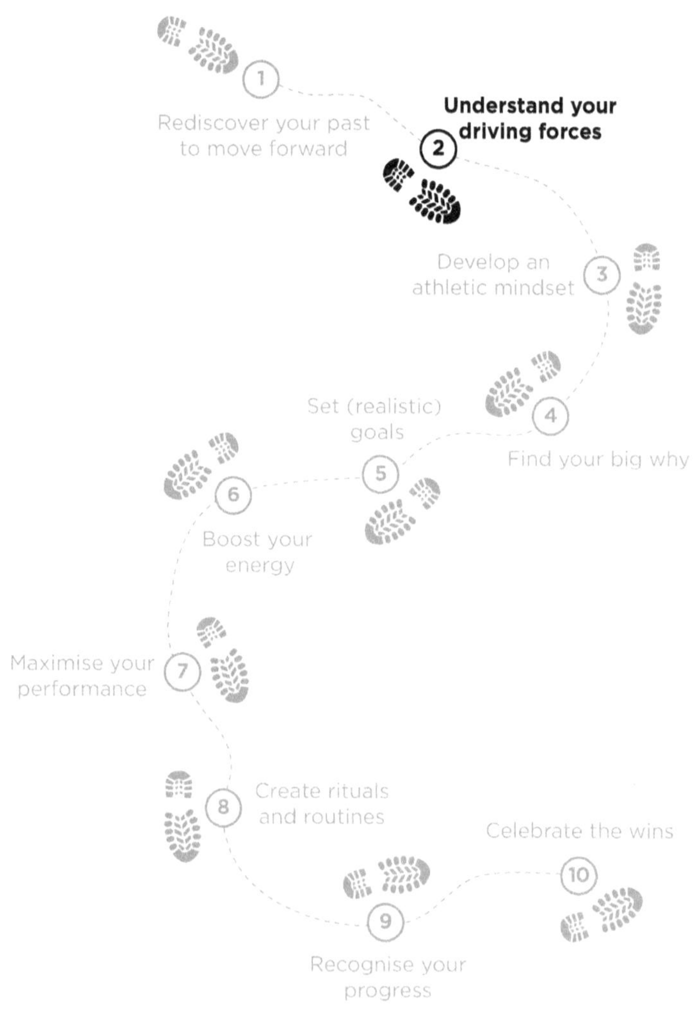

1
Rediscover your past to move forward
Understand your driving forces
2
Develop an athletic mindset
3
Set (realistic) goals
4
Find your big why
5
6
Boost your energy
Maximise your performance
7
Create rituals and routines
8
Celebrate the wins
10
9
Recognise your progress

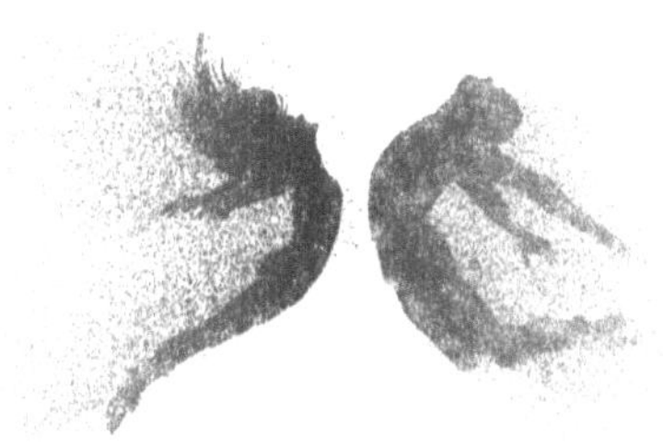

STEP 2:
UNDERSTAND YOUR DRIVING FORCES

So what happened back there in Step 1? I saw you – you started to smile and remember how excited you used to be. See it wasn't about time or effort, you were just in it, doing it. Well that old you is still in there somewhere. We just need to keep on digging.

So now you're starting to remember your Athlete Within. You're reconnecting to the good old days when you were that little ball of energy. Often we think we don't know where to start or what we need to do, yet our brains have a library of all our favourite stories of how we like to live our life. We just get caught up, thrown around, and forget to make the time to reflect.

Often our athletic ways are us following hunches, where we find enjoyment and freedom and want to be part of something just for the thrill of curiosity (what if I did this … ?).

Andrew didn't have anyone to drive him around from a very young age. If he wanted to go somewhere the easiest way was to just jump on his bike. He spent hours from morning to dark riding, finding the best fishing spots. The bike was his ticket to freedom.

At the end of our street, my friend had a long driveway and that meant only one thing: cricket. One of those old tin-can garbage bins for stumps that gave just the right sound when someone was bowled out. The rest is Australian history; our driveway was about being together. Everyone got to bowl, everyone got to bat, if the dog got your ball you were out, over the fence is six and out, fair and square.

Exercise

As you think back on the thing you loved doing the most, what made you do it? What was driving your Athlete Within?

WHAT PROPELS US

When was the last time you felt inspired, so inspired you could actually feel the excitement bubbling up inside you? What gets you out of bed? What gets you hungry *for change*? It could be knowing you are about to begin an adventure. Or an event, a special moment you know is coming. Or someone, or a thing, a feeling, a passion, a combination of everything you cherish in life: the big events dotted along the calendar and all the little things in between. You are the only one who knows what makes you tick.

To help you uncover what propels you, start by recognising and understanding where your energy is going. Our energy is spent on where we put our attention, something that can help us build our future or hold us back. And where our attention goes we find meaning. We attach meaning to our story, our thinking, and we become emotionally connected to that one thing. What propels us now has its reasons and we are connected to our big why.

What meaning and how much attention you want to give to what propels you is entirely up to you. Focusing on one thing directs greater energy to your reasons pushing you to jump into action, while spreading your attention over many things will dilute its power. Multitasking is often considered a very positive thing in our productivity-focused Western world, but in the quest to rediscover the Athlete Within it is something that we need to use sporadically.

Lisa has always considered herself the queen of multitasking. Yet when life doesn't follow the expected path, she can go into overdrive and feel overwhelmed. At those precise moments she gives attention to 'everything' on her plate: 'I'm late for work! I haven't exercised! There's nothing in the fridge!' She forgets to focus on the one thing that gives her pure joy and propels her forward: the love and pride she feels for the family she's built. Yes, she's running late for work but she's spending more time with the kids. She hasn't exercised but she can move when she walks around the block during a break. Dinner isn't ready yet but nobody is going to starve.

It's about deciding to give attention and meaning to the one thing that propels you. And when you make these decisions, in that exact moment you are defining what you desire and giving it priority. Our decisions propel and shape us, they separate not only us from each other but from who we are now and who we will be in the future. It is human nature to leave a decision at the door, till the final moment when the challenge or conflict becomes a crisis. The call to action is now. The more we take charge, find meaning and anticipate, the more we propel ourselves.

The more you understand the driving forces that propel your athlete within, the more hungry it gets and the more you can move forward and become it.

Exercise

What are three things you have been putting all your attention on?

Can you start to define three things that propel you forward?

Then can you find the one thing that these three have in common, the meaning?

Are you a multitasker? Peel it back and think about the thing you love doing the most and then think about why you give it priority.

YOUR MAGIC BOX

'In the midst of chaos there is opportunity.'

Sun Tzu

As we move deeper into your driving forces, it is time to look inside your magic box.

Why do you do some things but not others? Why are there times you hesitate, you don't follow through or you just talk yourself out of it before it even begins? Why is it that when you flip this, put yourself in the right frame of mind even in the face of a storm, you find your flow, you work your way through to the finish line? We can all show up with so much depth already inside us. Rediscovering your Athlete Within is about learning to use your magic box to tap into and find that something deeper within.

Your magic box is your art, the way you see the world, stirring it around with your past experiences, your beliefs, to give it your interpretation. Your magic box is a bank filled with strategies, the way you move through life, your challenges, your celebrations. And all you need is within this box. Standing guard at the door to your magic box takes patience, as does change. It is easy to slip back into old versions of ourselves, making choices that aren't congruent with who we are choosing to become.

The real question is: what has to happen for you to make changes? Our lives are full on. The pace is fast, there is a lot of noise, clutter, uncertainty, the push and the pull that at times feels like we are swimming non-stop just to keep above the water. In your magic box is your genius that you bring to the world, the way in which you operate, how you make sense of your environment.

In Step 2 we are breaking down your magic elements, how you filter incoming information, your beliefs, your finetuning processes and interpretations as well as interactions and feedback. Every 'training' session is an experiment, working with an idea, a deliberate intention, testing its effectiveness, honing in on the finer details until it feels right.

It is your magic box where you create the desires we call expectations and then compare them to what we believe is actually possible. Henry Ford famously said, 'whether you think you can or you think you can't – you're right'. Our magic box is the mix, the formulas, the way we put our world together both internally based on what we value as well as externally relative to our proximity and our mentors and role models. What has to happen for you to feel happy? Is there a number of ingredients, rules that have to be followed, hoops that have to be jumped through? Or is it just a matter of pausing to bring up a meaningful memory, a thought that makes you smile from the inside?

As you open your magic box, you are first going back in time and rediscovering your athletic self. This holds your key. More than just events, it harbours the feelings you associate, the steps that take place that engage you, the sequences that capture you which bring about your desired change from within. Teasing out this nitty gritty is your secret recipe. The more details you can decipher about your Athlete Within the more you draw it towards you.

Exercise

What holds value to you?

Are you using the tools in your magic box?

What has to happen or align in your life for you to make changes? Or to be happy?

What magic do you bring to the world? What's your art?

What details make your athlete within stand out even more?

IS IT TIME TO UPDATE YOUR BELIEFS?

Our beliefs are fiercely important. They are the way we see ourselves, the lens through which we read our story, the way we fit in, our vantage point relative to the rest of the world, our identity. Our beliefs are what we act out. Moving through life there are turning points where we learnt by just doing, where we built rules and strategies to create order. At the time they served a purpose, yet we carry the same beliefs with us now, holding onto what was. Recognising old beliefs that don't match or fit today's world means change – that requires courage and getting uncomfortable as we face the new. To shift our beliefs we have to break through our spell and return back to our magic box.

In her 20s Laura headed to the gym every afternoon following work. It made her feel healthy and like she was taking good care of herself. Starting a family brought all that to a grinding halt. Now in her 40s and with the kids grown up, she wants to get her old self back. It's just that the gym doesn't feel like *her* anymore, and has become more of a chore than something she enjoys. This leaves her feeling guilty, that she isn't doing the right thing for herself the way she used to. It's time to have a new conversation with herself, update some old beliefs and introduce the new version of Laura.

Daniel was a runner. He loved the feeling of freedom, being outdoors. In his 20s he enjoyed simply putting on his shoes and heading out for a run. But when his career took off, he put in more and more hours at the office and less on himself. A few promotions, a marriage and a young family changed his priorities. Fast forward to today, now in his 50s Daniel has a burning desire to relive that passion, popping on his new shoes and heading out for a run. A bit clanky and rusty at first, he has already found his old pace. Except that feeling of freedom he so wants to relive is just not there anymore. Even more crushing, he just doesn't like running anymore. And that's okay. It's time for Daniel to bring that sense of freedom into something new that he truly enjoys.

In Step 1 you revisited your past self and had a glimpse at some of the things you used to love doing as a little athlete. As we grow up, we learn more about what we like and how we make sense of what's around us. We develop a value system, a hierarchy of what we are attracted to and what we'd rather leave at the door. Often, with age, we take this a step further and we concentrate more on what we *don't* want than our desires.

In Step 2 you're asked to open up your magic box and start thinking about what you are attracted to, what you like and what your beliefs are now. Allow yourself to look inside your magic box to see what makes you *you*. Why do you love to cook, but hate the gym? Why is it you do not want go for a walk first thing in the morning but strolling along the beach on the weekend is something you love? Why is it you love playing tennis on holidays but when at home you would rather hang out on the couch and binge Netflix?

Exercise

What beliefs have you attached to the identity of your Athlete Within? Think about some of the rules and likes that have served you well in the past.

Can you identify beliefs that might be hindering your inner athlete or stopping you from being active now? Who would you need to be to see past these beliefs? What has to happen for you to become your Athlete Within?

MAKING CHANGE HAPPEN IN YOUR LIFE

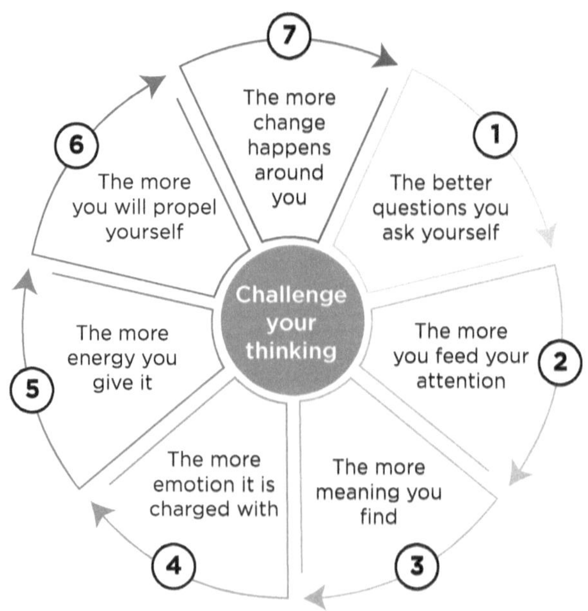

You're learning more and more about your beliefs and the meaning you give to everything in your life, your environment, what surrounds you. And you've probably identified some of the thinking that is holding you back from rediscovering your Athlete Within and moving to the next step. You can probably see some of the stories you tell yourself and the patterns you're stuck in – some of which we know are excuses. That's all actually pretty normal – everyone has stories that fit the way they feel and live. Change can be exciting and carry loads of energy back into your being, but change that brings purpose into your life can be challenging. And challenging yourself and your thinking is exactly what you need to do.

Once you start shifting some of these beliefs attached to your vision of your Athlete Within, you free up to see what you can become and your inner athlete can then truly take shape and come to life. When you change your thinking, you start asking yourself better questions, you put your attention to what has higher meaning to you and charge it with emotion. You give it energy and purpose, and you can then change. Habits tend to reinforce your thinking and beliefs, but by challenging the stories you tell yourself you can rewrite your story on your own terms.

So now is a good time to stop and spend some time (out of your usual environment) to challenge your thinking. If you continually improve the quality of your internal questions and work on your ability to make decisions, you propel yourself towards making change happen.

The thinking we do can hold us back. But it's also the way we associate feelings to past experiences and the way we talk to ourselves that can hinder our future. Think about the language you use when you talk about your Athlete Within. Are you encouraging or do you just talk yourself out of things easily? Think about how you feel in your body when you want to exercise but cannot be bothered. Even challenge the image you have of yourself as an athlete. These are all part of your beliefs that need a bit of a shakeup.

See, true change is driven by your ability to influence yourself, to turn your shoulds into musts. Influence is your ability to take charge of yourself (and your thinking) and lead, not just follow. It is about feeling excited, realising that everything resonates from the inside and you just need to take action. You become your own leader. You can get yourself up and over the threshold over and over, finding something so deep inside that it constantly drives you. And I can assure you anyone can do it. Anyone can be their own leader. Having an Athletic Mindset (Step 3) will help the process, but it's about being ready to challenge yourself and be creative when doing it. One step at a time.

At the end of the day, changing your thinking is about making your stories a little bit easier. Getting rid of the roadblocks that stop you. Let go of the rules by going through them one at a time. Ultimately it comes from within but there are ways you can help shape who you want to become by working on your proximity, by changing your environment. Lisa loves fresh blooms, so on Fridays, just before karate, she goes around the block to pick some flowers to put in a vase to encourage herself to change and go to training, just go for it. What you create around you can have an incredible influence, and sooner or later also help you find that influence inside of you so you can propel forward on your own two feet.

Exercise

How would you need to change your thinking to let your Athlete Within come to the surface? Do you need to look at the way you talk to yourself? The stories you tell yourself? Can you go a bit easier on yourself?

Can you change something around you to help you bring change inside of you?

When you think about your Athlete Within, do you feel it in your body? Does the thought leave you feeling tired, unenthusiastic and upset? Or does it fill you with energy, move you, and make you want to stand tall with readiness?

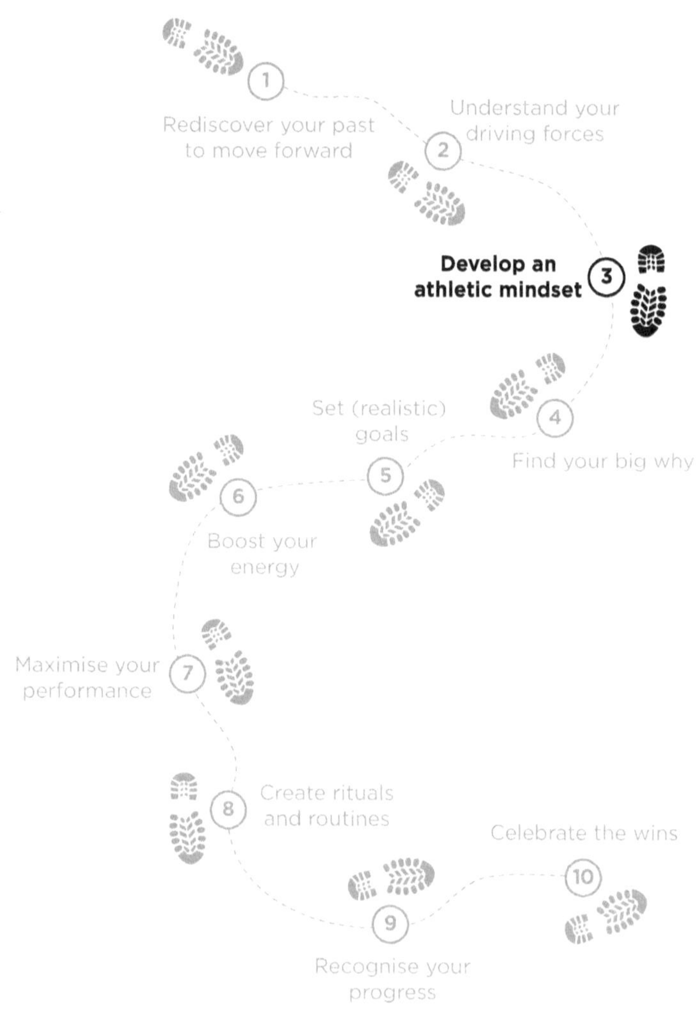

1
Rediscover your past to move forward
2
Understand your driving forces
Develop an athletic mindset 3
4
Find your big why
Set (realistic) goals
5
6
Boost your energy
7
Maximise your performance
8
Create rituals and routines
Celebrate the wins
10
9
Recognise your progress

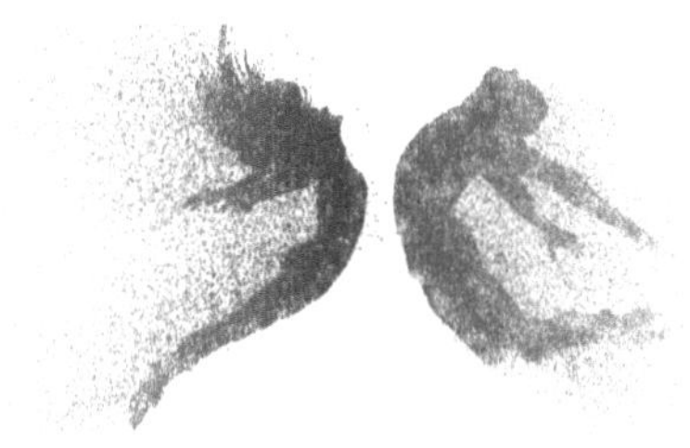

STEP 3:
DEVELOP AN ATHLETIC MINDSET

WHAT IS AN ATHLETIC MINDSET?

We have just spent some time uncovering your driving forces, understanding that some old beliefs, habits and values may need to change. Think about it a bit like a spring clean. Now it's time to go a step further and make sure you're equipped with the right tools to rediscover your Athlete Within.

An athletic mindset is made up of an inner core, shaped by you, and an outer shell, shaped by the world around you.

Your inner core

Your inner core is made out of **grind**, **grit** and **growth**. It is the internal dialogue, your internal map, that begins with the way you operate from the inside. It is the result of honing over time, dedication and nurturing towards mastery. The aim of the inner core is to work till it becomes a part of you, so you can last the distance. It is how you dedicate your life towards the long haul. It is more than a one-trick wonder; it has authenticity, endurance (longevity) and can stand adversity. The most amazing part of your inner core is your ability to influence yourself, to become your own athlete, your own leader.

Your Athlete Within is a place where you aren't following the crowd, you are running your own race, you are staying in your own lane. Who you are is defined by your own standards you set, your own definition at your own pace. It is when you draw a line in the sand and you begin to enter your internal world and play the internal game at your own level.

Your outer shell

The outer shell of mindset is made out of **mentors**, **proximity** (what's close to us) and **accountability**. It is what you learn from the world around you, watching how people interact, discussing ideas with your tribal members, seeking words of wisdom in an effort to better yourself at your athletic endeavour. These voices are important to your inner athlete as they are an outside opinion; they are resources that provide perspective but also insight from their library of knowledge and experience.

Whether they are words from a coach or a mentor, these are the people who are your guides along the way. Learning is a many-pronged beast, and it can be difficult to be vulnerable, take advice or try something different. It opens your eyes, recalibrates your lens and can only expand your game towards mastery.

When you reach clarity around all aspects of the athletic mindset you set yourself up for success and truly understand how to become your Athlete Within.

*

The athletic mindset is about understanding where your attention flows and refocusing or recalibrating. It is understanding that our minds drift into different scenarios, acting out different events, playing different strategies from different angles to find the solution that fits. It is also realising that our minds can easily move from feelings of elation to deflation, especially when we are trying to start something new (like rediscovering the Athlete Within). We may become frustrated or anxious, thinking that our minds should be driven in a straight line, carrying on like work horses with blinkers. Yet our minds are adventurous, built to forage, seek adventure and mull over a problem with the freedom to create. Our mind loves meandering, zigzagging, curving and even going backwards.

Our mindset is shaped from the day we are born. We have inherent biases we carry with us from our upbringing and we then add our own experiences, past attempts and results into the mix, essentially forming our learnings. We then blend these lessons with our current views we call perception; how we see the everyday of our world unfolding. We complete our view of the world by sprinkling some rules on top, just for added complexity.

Our version of life exists somewhere along the gap between perception and expectation: the larger the gap, the more unhappiness and uneasiness we tend to experience. As if our own internal labyrinth wasn't enough to unscramble, our focus is often drawn to the outer world where we begin to measure and compare ourselves to others, widening that gap further. We are trying to make sense of the order and chaos that exists around us in our outer world that is ultimately incongruent with our inner environment.

To move forward we require an understanding of what forms our mindset and the willingness to move past our current version, taming our mind through the art of deliberate focus.

In rediscovering your athlete, it is your mindset that begins setting the bar and determining your beliefs on what is actually possible.

It's important to spend some time understanding how you see yourself, the world, and yourself in this world as mindset can truly be the make or break of what we start, how far we follow through and whether we make it to the finish line.

Exercise

Consider the way you think and how you approach the world.

How wide is the gap between your reality and your expectations? What is one thing you can tackle to start narrowing that gap and become more in tune with your Athlete Within?

GRIND

'Just do it.'

Nike

Grind is just starting and then doing the work. It's where we make it happen. We implement our decisions, we take immediate action, we demonstrate 'we can' and it is game on. Grind is the effort we put in.

The challenge of the first step

Often people become confused and discouraged when taking the first step, feeling it needs to be grand, and as a result it often is the hardest part. The reality is starting is just new, raw and clumsy. We kinda know that getting started is the first test along the journey, but we might not be aware that to truly set off we need to make a pact with ourselves, reach a threshold and step into the now towards a new tomorrow.

Not born with the greatest of anatomical equipment, Lisa was plagued with injuries in her youth, attempting sport that led her to surgery trying to rectify congenital disadvantages. Her father, in his quest to help his daughter, introduced her to karate to help her better understand her body mechanics, and in so doing set her on a journey of physical but also self-discovery. Today, well into her 40s, she is a mum, a businesswoman and the wearer of many more hats. Working on her athletic mindset, Lisa immediately recognised her difficulty at starting. Even though she loves karate and is longing to rekindle her relationship with the sport to improve her physicality, she keeps finding reasons why she can't. A lot of her story lies in her external world. With a 15-year-old son plus six-year-old twins, every day is an adventure, dancing with busyness that keeps taking her away from herself and into the external. She finds it easier to focus on what everyone else needs and put herself last, pointing to her never-ending to-do list, giving her reasons or something to blame, tangled in her own web of procrastination.

How often do we find ourselves starting and stopping, going through the cycles and turnstiles of life? Just like a New Year's Eve resolution, we often start looking for our Athlete Within with the best intentions, yet without following a process and building our story, the wheels soon fall off as the chaos of life flows back in.

Lisa is stuck, handbrake on.

Hitting the grind unlocks the handbrake

Once we get going, there's a period where we are just learning the ropes, becoming familiar with what we're doing, building awareness and intelligence, and working our way up to game level. Often it's not till we are 'in it' that we appreciate the fullness of what's involved.

Some people, like me, love the grind. It's putting in the grunt, testing yourself against some struggle, pushing the edge, knowing that at the end you will be that little bit closer. We live on the side of a mountain with which I have developed a relationship, just because it's there (it speaks to me). When I mention this to other people, there are some who look at me and nod, knowing – and then there are others who just look at me, eyes wide. Walking the trail that winds up this mountain has turned into running that has now turned into lengthening and exploring other hills. Growing up I always had a knack for hills. There is something about digging your toes in and doing the work required to get to the top. Pushing through the physical demands, the pleading emotions, the ability to grind the mountain till I reach the top.

Doing the work of the Athlete Within means embracing many different aspects such as discipline, technique, motivation – all elements I cover in this book. For the time being though, think of grind as the effort you put in, your own way to work the physical to build the mental. When you *do* (and keep doing) you *become*.

A key element in rediscovering your Athlete Within is to look back at your experiences to find your own answers – how you have dealt with a similar situation before. If we have already faced it, chances are we understand what is required and who we have to become to move forward.

Exercise

Go back to a time when you told yourself 'I can do it' and you succeeded. What did it feel like? What made you say 'yes!'? What did you enjoy about the grind?

And if you think starting is difficult, what reasons do you tell yourself why 'you can't'? What permission do you need to give yourself to 'just do it'?

GRIT

Grit, simply put, is what keeps us going. What truly drives people to do more, become more and break barriers. How about you – what is it that gets you excited, fired up, drawn to something bigger and makes you carry on?

There is a lot of research into grit, particularly by psychologist and popular science author Angela Duckworth, who aligns grit with perseverance. Grit is continuing to work for a period of time, sticking it out until we complete the game.

Julian is high up in the corporate world of law. At the turning point of 40, he finds himself overweight, overtired and living with pain. Used to the everyday work grind and wired to find solutions, he decides to reignite his passion for running and get on top of his health. Beginning with walking along bush trails near his house, he enjoys following the process and finding his way back into running. He finds pleasure in being physical again and keeps taking steps towards change, rediscovering his own Athlete Within, slowly increasing the kilometres and making the time to build his training.

Over the months, he decides he wants to fulfil a long-lost dream of running a marathon. He chooses a particular event to steer his training towards. Being a great lawyer, he knows he needs a deadline.

The three months before the event require a lot more effort from Julian to find time to train, among work requirements and the needs of his young family. But he is no stranger to hard work and persever-ance. He counts down the days as he racks up his training kilometres. He completes the event with enthusiasm, proudly showing his finish-ing medal to anyone interested (I was). He moves smoothly into his recovery training and starts talking about the marathon he wants to do the following year. Julian moves easily into grind and it's almost a natural step into grit, embracing the push of will to reach a high achievement. It's all about the goal.

Grit begins deep inside

But there is more to grit than a desire to achieve and finish. Grit is something that begins deep on the inside, right down in your belly. It's a human characteristic, a part of our survival. Inside each of us there is more than even we realise – the well goes deep.

Angela Duckworth describes passion as a key quality in grit, but what is passion?

Passion is an internal inspiration, your reason for doing things; it is pure, it is authentic and it pulls you from within. Passion is more than the goals you set yourself to achieve. It is the reason you achieve them. It is the reason that will stay with you and will push you to continue being your Athlete Within well after you've reached your goals.

Julian really wants to do that second marathon, but with time he loses enthusiasm, anticipation and fulfilment, and the running comes to a grinding halt. Life has taken over. More than that, he understands that moving from one deadline to the next (one marathon to another) can certainly help develop grit, but to truly become the Athlete Within the doing and the perseverance need to turn into growth, a way of life.

Finding your grit is a key turning point in developing your athletic mindset to stand the test of time. It is upon grit we build momentum and start reaping the rewards, where the learnings become our wisdom.

Exercise

Think of grit as the fuel to your aspirations and desires – can you remember a time when you were in the grit and enjoying the process? How did it feel? What did you like or dislike? Did 'carrying on' come easy to you? What was the reason behind your grit?

And how about now – do you have grit? If not, what perceptions and beliefs can you work on to change this? How can you turn it into your best ally?

GROWTH

'A ship in harbour is safe, but that is not what ships are built for.'

Author John A. Shedd

Julian did run that first marathon and achieve his goal, but he stopped at the second one. He just couldn't do it. His Athlete Within was probably a bit bored, not really keen to do the work again. He had plateaued and couldn't carry on – grind and grit were not enough. What Julian lacked was *growth*. Along the way to running his first major event he definitely learned lessons, and acquired essential knowledge and understanding of himself and how he tackled challenges. What growth does though is make you stop and use that knowledge – to look at your current situation and reassess and find a way forward. Growth is understanding you have reached a plateau – physical (I can't run anymore) or emotional (I just don't have it in me) – and allowing yourself to change things up so you break your ceiling and find your next level. Your Athlete Within becomes part of your life; being active is what you do regardless. It's who you are.

Growth is an essential part of your Athlete Within. It comes from the deepest part of your inner being. Growth is an approach, a way of thinking, of not getting caught by the tentacles of the world but feeling freedom instead. It is here we unleash, let go, become creative, try new things and tap into our true athlete. It is setting new expectations and testing them against the environment, challenging the world – why do things need to be this way?

Embrace change

When you grow you feel you are working with change, sensing a forward progression, knowing you are riding the wave of momentum.

Growth is letting go and letting life unfold so you can become more, revealing your true nature. In a nutshell, a growth mindset is how we deal with failure – the process of learning. This is a concept that has been investigated in fascinating detail by author and researcher Carol Dweck.

What if Julian, faced with a second marathon, adjusted his target rather than trying to repeat what he had just achieved (and clearly felt proud about)? He knew 'he could' run the whole 42 km, so what elements of that win could he use and apply to something else? Maybe even to a much smaller feat, one that he could access easily, one that still reminded him that 'he could', one that still made him proud of himself and to feel he 'did it'. Growth is the ability to relive the feelings of our successes and rewards, and taking these experiences out of our heads and into our body, our hearts. It fuels the way of life of the Athlete Within.

Craig, a very successful businessman, visited my clinic at regular intervals for more than 10 years – making sure his body was keeping up as he aged was a very important part of his beliefs. He knew that if he 'serviced it' regularly just like a car, he would have many years of life ahead to enjoy, for himself and his young son. Having grown up enjoying athletics as a teenager within a sporting family, he particularly re-embraced the importance of physicality and condition in his 60s during his own pursuit of rediscovering his Athlete Within.

He was a planner, and scheduled being active into his agenda just as he would an important meeting. Craig was also a realist, continually recalibrating relative to the phase of life he was in.

The growth phase of rediscovering your Athlete Within is a progressive pursuit of learning and adapting. It is about integrating; taking on board the lessons and making sure they become a part of the way we live our life for the long haul. In growth we transform from 'I can' to 'I own it', where an ability we pursue and nourish becomes mastery.

Exercise

Think about how you store your experiences in your memory bank. Do you go back and learn from them? Are you able to apply the lessons to whatever you are facing now? How do you tackle boredom? What is it that makes you grow?

*

FIND YOUR MENTORS

A mentor is someone you can draw inspiration from, often bringing clarity and wisdom to the table. A mentor is someone you trust and admire as they are true masters of their art, and you hang on their every word hoping to soak up some of their knowledge, their cool, their mastery.

For your Athlete Within, mentors can be a catalyst.

First of all, mentors are 'outside your game' – they are not in the heat of your grind, so they can provide a comforting and inspiring voice from their vantage point. Often when you're 'in it' you can't find a solution or a way forward, even if it's right in front of you. Mentors don't hold all the answers and they certainly don't have a crystal ball, but we appreciate the importance of looking at things from a different angle.

Mentors are people you trust because they've been where you are now and they've learned lessons they can share. They provide a point of reference and security we can use to pull ourselves forward. Hundreds of thousands of years ago young athletes would have approached the elders, those with experience, connected to earlier times, and would have soaked up stories and anecdotes to help them make sense of the road ahead.

Mentors become people you lean on because they are in your corner. They take time to get to know you, to understand what ticks your boxes. They sense and show you what you're capable of, they listen, make you feel special, they encourage you to expand and bring out the best in you. They are part of your A-team. At the end of the day, you had mentors from the moment you were born: your parents. Starting us on our way, they were making the best decisions available to them with what they were equipped for at the time, the goal being to provide security, love and happiness.

As we progress through life we also draw inspiration and understanding from others: teachers, coaches, older siblings or other family members, as well as cultural influences. Picking your mentors is one part innocence (what we inherently feel supports us) and one part knowledge of yourself (what we have grown to know works).

Your mentors may provide unparalleled insight, but ultimately only you can decide how to use it.

Exercise

Think about the mentors around you who are in your corner no matter what. Is there anyone you can approach right now to add to your A-team as a resource, someone to bounce ideas off or help you look for what's possible? Who could be your greatest mentor and inspiration?

What if you needed a new mentor? What would they look like? How would they help you in your journey of rediscovery?

WHAT'S GOING ON AROUND YOU?

'With the knowledge you've been given, you are now on the inside of what I like to call … "the Byrnes family circle of trust."'

Jack Byrnes, *Meet the Fockers*

From the moment you wake, your brain starts taking everything in, putting on the radar, becoming alert and making sense of the world around you. Like a Terminator, you scan the landscape, zoning in and registering particular objects (don't step on that Lego piece left on the floor!), you interpret and process everything. Your brain makes sense of what's around you.

Then in comes the phone with the socials, the news feed and the reminders. Suddenly your brain starts thinking about the email you haven't written, the phone call with the accountant to organise the taxes, the pile of clothes you still haven't put away, the lunchboxes to fill, the drycleaning to pick up. You get out of bed and your mind is already full to the brim because now you've added your emotions, your tiredness and your frustrations to your environment and 'ouch', you step on that Lego piece and it hurts, but not as much as the back that has been giving you grief for a while.

All this stuff, these meanings, these piles, become your context. And context is your proximity.

Proximity

When my wife is happy she is singing, dancing and arranging flowers around the house – the message is clear. The kitchen is usually tidy, there is some order around her and she doesn't feel the stress of deadlines. It is also very clear when she wakes up a fiery dragon, set alight by the toys scattered around the house or the dirty dishes in the sink, but I'd better not get into that or I'll end up incinerated.

Our world is our orbit. What moves around us we attract and become attracted to – it's the pull. Who you are depends very much on how you're tuned in to what's inside and outside of you. Proximity is the world you inhabit and what you have built around you. Your proximity can be an ally but also a trap, boxing you in, keeping you from growing. When we are struggling, we feel heavy, exhausted, not in our element. There are piles of unfinished tasks building up, the house always feels untidy, the kids unruly and things increase in complexity. Low priorities fill up the void. On the other end, when we're tuned in and aligned with ourselves, in purpose, everything seems to work in unison and the day becomes one to remember and cherish.

Entrepreneur, author and motivational speaker Jim Rohn challenges us: 'Show me the top five books you are reading, the key five people in your life and I will tell you who you will be and the life you will be living in five years' time.'

That rings so true. When I listen to my clients I can always tell where they're at and what's happening in their proximity because the topics will always flow to what has substance and meaning to them. I can quickly discover where their heart is and their passion just by listening to where they light up in the conversation. Proximity shows us what we value.

Proximity is an often underestimated player when it comes to building an athletic mindset because we do not always know we have some control over it. We can actually work on it, improve it and model it to support our Athlete Within and help us succeed. We can shape the world around us and keep the things we like, that build us up, that help us grow and make us feel good because, as self-help author and speaker Anthony Robbins puts it, 'Where focus goes, energy flows'. Buddha echoes the feeling by reminding us that 'what we think, we become'.

Your proximity is made out of everything around you; it can be a person, a thing, a trend, an idea. It includes what you think about yourself, the people around you, the community you live in and how you fit in. As social animals, we are very influenced by what is around us. We are very aware of the games and hierarchy playing out and we have a strong desire to be part of something bigger. The people in your inner circle are your influencing group and they are also your comparison group – how you measure yourself.

Exercise

So now think about your proximity. Physically, what can you change to set yourself up for success? What are simple steps you can take (one at a time) to make the environment around you a place that influences you for the best? Where do you spend your time, and where do you put your attention?

On an emotional level, are the people in your proximity stretching and encouraging you or setting you back? How do you feel when you think about them? And how about your community? Do you feel supported? Understood? Are there groups around you that can help you lift up?

ACCOUNTABILITY

'A chain is only as strong as its weakest link.'

Philosopher Thomas Reid

The people who hold you accountable are the ones who help you grow into your own master. They don't fear the opponent, there's no competition, they have perspective and they are able to give the honesty you need and you can rely on. At times they are your confidantes, your right hand, your best resource. Accountability is about choosing who you let into your team, your A-team, your partners in crime, the wing-people who help you increase your chances of becoming your Athlete Within.

Just showing up is a huge step forward in rediscovering your Athlete Within, yet often we fall back into our habits and what we know. Change can be hard. This is where your accountability buddy becomes your biggest asset and steps in to save the day. It feels amazing when you have the support of someone, when a person you trust and admire tells you that you can go another step. They encourage you for just getting out there even if it is snowing, or they celebrate with you because you hit a milestone, no matter how small it may seem.

When we get challenged we can shrink, look for a corner or talk our way out of it. But your accountability buddy, or even your coach, is on your side. They don't give up on you, they understand the long game and they believe in you. They are a powerful resource in managing all the tricky steps and obstacles you may need to negotiate, strategically working through the challenges, your greatest spectators cheering you on from the sideline. Often your accountability buddy becomes a great part of your life, someone you can lean on, talk to, a true friend as you now have a shared history.

What is key in setting up accountability is going through the rules of engagement. What is involved in the relationship? What structure is in place, setting boundaries and metrics or milestones to meet along the way? Picking your team is often harder than we think, yet done well, it increases your chances of success. There are some who like to go alone, the lone wolves among us, which is okay. We all have to do what works for us. Yet working with a buddy or tribe can create a stronger meaning, more pull, a force to be reckoned with. A buddy can be your shadow, see another way in or around or even just be your support, your greatest fan. It plays out in many ways.

Exercise

Following on from defining proximity, now think about who is in your current A-team. Are they there for the right reasons? Are they a sounding board? Are they honest, direct, authentic? If you're about to create your A-team, what rules and milestones do you need to set upfront to get the most out of accountability? And if you are indeed a lone wolf, how do you stay accountable?

DEALING WITH SETBACKS AND OBSTACLES

We all have to deal with obstacles and setbacks. In many ways, it is how we learn. Having practised in the heart of the city, I have had the good fortune to work with the elite in business, politics and sports, seeing firsthand how they approach the world around them, what mindset they adopt in a tricky situation (they were after all dealing with a very real injury or chronic pain). Some worked within strict guidelines, their rules of engagement, getting in and out, a very clear and clinical interaction. Others had different approaches, sometimes appearing slow, more cognitive, in some ways harder to work with. One ex Australian Prime Minister had the tendency to repeat back to me what we were working with, something I found incredibly intimidating: 'If I understand you correctly, this is what the problem is and this is the way we are going about it.'

I realised that when I worked with such people I was stepping into their world and glancing directly into their mindset. They were defining what the problem was in the moment, laying out options and why we decided to work in that way and their expected outcomes. At the end they would ask, *how did we go today, was this what we wanted?*

Early on I was overplaying it, thinking they were challenging my work. But they were just being interactive and defining their expectations against their target goal. In the end, I really enjoyed working with them and looked forward to their appointments.

Having the privilege of going along my clients' journeys, I have come to learn that a lot of the time people already know the answer to their problems, they just make it more complex than it needs to be. There's a question I like to ask myself when I encounter an obstacle: 'How much can I learn about this scenario in this moment?' It forces me to read each situation as it is. It isn't about blowing it up and making it bigger than what it is, nor getting stuck in a cycle. It begins with where we are standing (define the problem) at this moment and what is in front of us or ahead along the way (anticipation). Then it's down to the decisions we take.

This is when you can dip into your athletic mindset. There isn't a right recipe you can use to solve problems but more of a personal mix of all the elements of your inner core and outer shell. The solution could be lying in any of those areas. When you are plateauing, you can look at growth and see how you can challenge yourself more. If you injure yourself you can go to your A-team and seek help. When you lack motivation you could look at your proximity to find inspiration and a push.

We have had to face obstacles and setbacks from the very first moment we entered this world. How you deal with them is what sets your Athlete Within apart. Having a big reason to move forward and help you navigate the hard bits is also key to your success and that's where we're heading to in the next step, but for the time being there's only one thing I want you to remember and that is that everything you need to overcome is right there, inside of you.

Exercise

Think about how you deal with problems. Do you fall into a heap and get overwhelmed or do you tackle them straight on? What do you tell yourself?

Do you have an analytical approach to problem solving or more a 'wing it' mentality?

Next time you are stuck, first define the problem: where are you at in this point in time?

What is the setback or obstacle? Is it tangible? Can you measure it? Can you anticipate the bumps on the road?

Are you reading the situation in the right way? What is another approach you could explore?

ALL YOU NEED IS IN YOU

In Step 1 you went into your past to uncover your present and unlock your future. You followed your trail back.

In Step 2 you examined your beliefs to understand more of you.

In Step 3 you are now the apprentice on your way to mastery, realising that all you need is indeed in you. You are leading your Athlete Within. It is about becoming resourceful and understanding how to influence yourself to take action.

Knowing that whatever happens you are resourceful, you are not afraid of making the important decisions, the path ahead is not always the easy road but you are prepared to take on its challenges. With this mindset you bravely step forward, into the unknown, and become someone you are proud of, you are able, you know it is just a continuation of moving forward, of following the process, of growing by staying on the path.

Why? Because it's an internal thing, it's your essence, it's who you truly are, it is a calling from somewhere deep inside. Something that resonates with you, something that has meaning for you, something that will give you a feeling of fulfilment and strength.

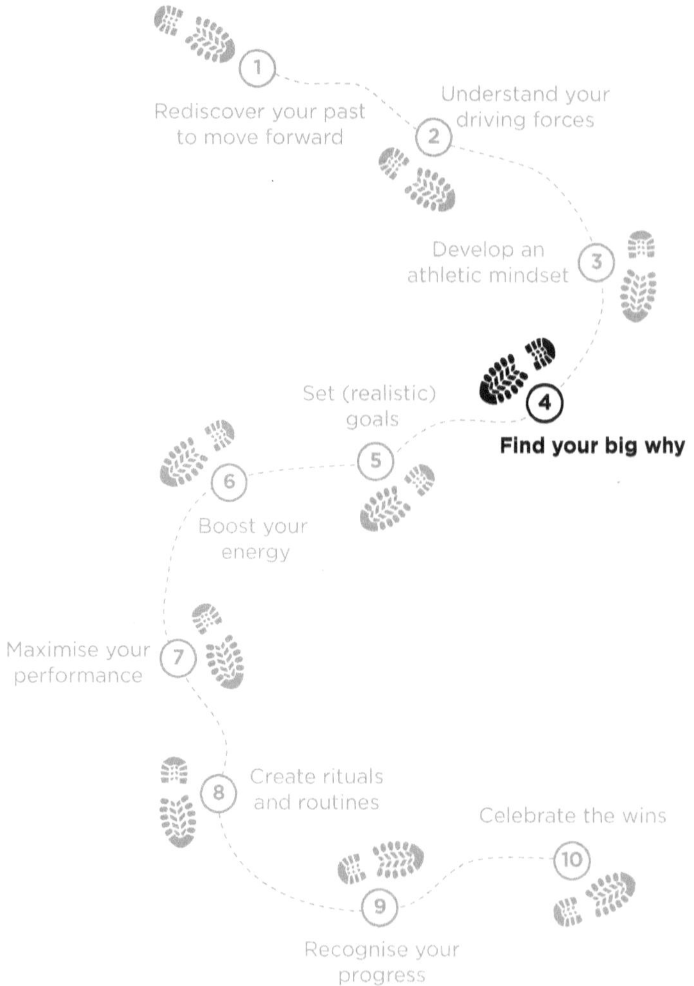

1
Rediscover your past to move forward
2
Understand your driving forces
3
Develop an athletic mindset
4
Find your big why
5
Set (realistic) goals
6
Boost your energy
7
Maximise your performance
8
Create rituals and routines
9
Recognise your progress
10
Celebrate the wins

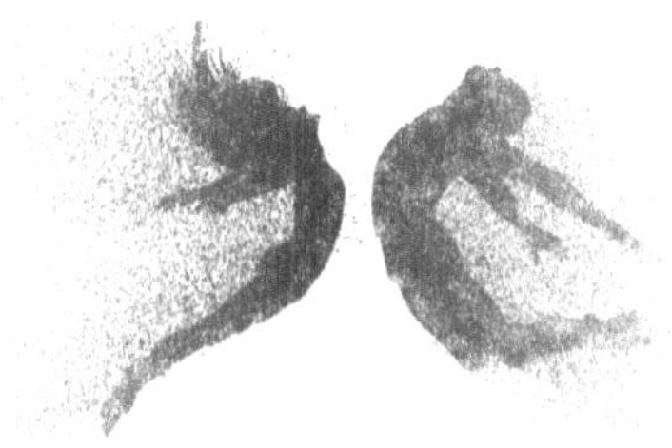

STEP 4:
FIND YOUR BIG WHY

START WITH THE BIGGER PICTURE

With the knowledge you now have about what makes an athletic mindset, and in particular what can push you to grow and overcome obstacles and setbacks, you can now move into the next step of your journey of rediscovery.

Few of us truly contemplate the bigness of life. It's easier to be swept up in the day to day which feels important, but meaning comes with perspective, so let's start with the bigger picture. Becoming and knowing are key parts to your bigger journey, the way you approach your overarching question of life. Knowing what drives you is liberating, it gives you depth, humility and gratitude through understanding. It is this perspective that gives you freedom. The day to day takes on a different shape.

We all have our calling, that drive inside. Take the time to listen to it, become familiar with it and nurture it, and grow.

Who are you?

What makes you *you*?

What is important to you?

Why?

But why?

But why?

Find one thing

Pick one thing.

Why does it mean so much to you?

What do you think about that deepens this feeling?

What is the biggest part of this, your why?

What about it penetrates so deep inside you, that brings up your emotions?

How would you describe this why?

There are times in life you feel a deeper sense of something, you just can't put your finger on it but it just feels so right. It connects, it resonates, it speaks to you and takes you further. There is no textbook, a way that is right. It is your internal knowing that is talking.

Reconnecting with your Athlete Within is looking inside at what resonates, what is meaningful, and deciding why we do what we do. Essentially the reasons that will drive you come first, make you hungry, leave you wanting more, then the answers come second. Yet we get caught up in our own story, tied up by our own rules and way of life. Is your story more of an internally or externally driven scenario? Are you looking for achievement, recognition or glory, or are you trying to find meaning, a way of feeling about yourself? As you start to see your own story in this light, it will already be guiding you towards your own why.

Uncovering your why is digging around inside to find your own truth; for some this is an inner calling, for others just a strong sense of purpose. A strong *why root* is found by asking questions until you feel it deep in your belly, it resonates and pulls you, you feel hot or cold, there is a knowing that this is right. Like a thread, when you start pulling you begin to untangle more. It is about trusting the process of rediscovering your Athlete Within.

When I work one on one with people we talk about the 'ultimate upsetter'. In life we tend to hold beliefs on how the world should be, often tying ourselves to one position that we start to defend. Freedom comes when you can see what you are attached to, what you think you can't do without. Breaking free means uncovering your ultimate upsetter. More than often this is moving from a place in your head to rediscovering a place in your heart. This can trigger a domino effect, like opening a door to understanding, realising you have been doing it one way, the same way, all this time, but now there is a new way. It just means letting go.

In the age of social media, there are many stories of people pushing against the odds, having braved serious accidents, financial ruin or other significant life events.

These people have all faced a moment of monumental decision, pressured by the ticking of time and adversity requiring an immediate re-evaluation of what is significant to them at that one moment. We are drawn to their stories of becoming something more than who they are in that moment, perhaps sensing their calling or demand to be something greater, the way they found a way to pull through. Yet at the same time it can leave one feeling our own personal story lacking, that it doesn't have the value or isn't as important.

The truth is each of us carries our own why story for our Athlete Within. Often clouded by time, we work towards understanding life, grasping meaning between chaos and order to find our place. Underneath our expectations of how the world works and our perceptions that form our reality, we each hold reasons, our *why root*.

Exercise

What is the story you are telling yourself about your own why?

What is your why root?

THE FIERCE URGENCY OF NOW

It's easy to think 'one day'. One day I will … ? But what? *What* will you do one day? Distraction is putting it off till tomorrow, telling yourself 'you can't', training yourself 'you can't'.

Let's brainstorm this feeling, grab it by the horns and give it a big shake. Think back to your dream list – when are you going to go after it? When is a good time? Stop and pick one thing. What is that one thing on your list? Before you ask, 'can I do this?', or, 'how will I do this?' – pull back and think '*why* should I do this?' All the clues are there – the breadcrumb trail leads back to your why. How will it serve me, fulfill me, expand who I am?

Your mind doesn't want to get out of bed, it's going to be too cold, it's still dark, you don't know what you are going to wear today. 'Why' is waking your mind up, asking the 'why' question again and again to cut through the layers until you get to your *why root*.

As humans our evolutionary brilliance comes in the form of thinking. Just like a time capsule, we can travel back and live in the past or we can propel ourselves forward and play out the future, be our own devil's advocate or find possibilities, another way forward. At the same time we can be our own worst enemies, getting stuck in our heads, not ever actually moving forward, being lost in our illusion. Just like Walter Mitty, we can run off in our heads and save a dog from a building on fire, the hero in our own imaginary world. But as the movie progresses, imagination moves into reality and Walter finishes the movie a true hero.

For a lot of us, rediscovering the Athlete Within may begin in our heads, but taking the first step means making decisions and taking action. Living life is about pulling your attention in, making a decision and taking action with what is in front of you in this moment.

Thinking about now is about giving you a starting point, being decisive, stepping out of hesitation and frustration and writing down your why root. Your why root may be a thread that when you start to pull it is attached to something bigger, and soon you find yourself in the fabric of who you are. Often I advise people to keep hold of their why root for a period of six months, then actively revisit it. With growth our why root may expand, go deeper, and we may start to shift our direction. But make the decision now and move forward with a strong root to hold on to.

OWN IT

Constantly pushing your why root further and further away is a form of procrastination, moving to a place just out of reach. A place where you can then add in all those other stories of 'why not'. Rather than believe, you may like to confuse, average things out and cause distraction. It may feel more satisfying at first to work on many things, building piles of unfinished plans around you. It could bring feelings of importance, of significance. But these fun distractions are only short lived and not overly fulfilling.

Owning your why root is key for the Athlete Within. Owning it means rehearsing it and developing a deeper relationship with your why root. As a test, if someone woke you at 3 am and you could move back into the feeling of your why, it is then that you know you own it. Just like every relationship, your Athlete Within takes time and commitment. Even with the right why root, it still needs attention and work.

A key part to owning your why root is in anticipation. We all know what it feels like when we finally approach an event or something we've been waiting for. The build up is palpable and as we get closer we get more and more excited. Anticipation brings us into the moment and takes the feeling – the why root – out of our head and into our heart and body.

> **Exercise**
>
> What is a question you could ask yourself every morning to engage the feeling of your why root? Could you build anticipation into the question?

IS YOUR WHY BIG ENOUGH?

When a ship is built, it is tested to survive the harshest of conditions, when the ocean is at its wildest and most unpredictable. When the ship is being tossed and thrown around, through it all it comes out on top. What is inside you? What are you built for?

You may choose to train towards a big adventure like a marathon, which inherently requires patience and pacing yourself to build the ability and intelligence required. At a higher level, you don't want to become a one-hit wonder and fall back to your starting point, a roller-coaster ride that puts your body under more havoc and drives you further away from your why.

Julian has discovered his why root, realising a marathon was a fixed challenge – for him it was the equivalent of traveling into space … tick, but … what next? Keep upping the ante. You have to keep feeding the beast, either go bigger or go home.

Is your why root big enough to stretch you? Is it a why root that can take you further, take you out of the comfort zone, give you the opportunity to change who you are, deep enough to pull you through, overcome the conditions you face and grow?

Alan loved competing in Ironman races. He had a strong healthy why root, yet with a growing young family and a demanding work schedule, his training was disciplined but was inconsistent. Through the years he kept his sight on the bigger picture, participating in at least two triathlons per year, occasionally more. After about six years the kids were older, his job changed to one requiring no travel – a tipping point. He had his chance. Dedicating a room to training, he increased his capacity and his consistency. His why root had stood the test of time. Progressively he applied himself, accrued the required points over a two-year period and achieved his childhood dream: a chance to compete in the world-famous Hawaiian triathlon.

Exercise

Is your why root big enough when it comes to your Athlete Within? Will it stand the test of time?

Are you stepping away from comfort?

Are you challenging your rules and beliefs on how your Athlete Within should be?

Will it stretch you, ask you to be more, greater than where you are at the moment, and change you towards growth?

MAKE IT YOURS

A researcher who used to see me in the clinic was filled with a strong passion to understand cancer, having lost her mum to the disease when she was a child. It meant long hours for years in a lab, often with small breakthroughs. She held onto big ideas for where she felt the answers lay. The flipside of this was she loved to run. There were times when work and family were intense; her running never stopped, she just reined it in to fit with her life. Sometimes she would run at night, shorter distances as it was late, but she enjoyed and soaked up the cooler air, the quietness of her neighbourhood. For some reason, running at night allowed her to think things through; not just the challenges faced each day, but turning her attention towards her bigger questions. She shared that sometimes she felt her mum running beside her, and that in those moments she experienced calmness and a deeper passion for life. She later remembered that when she was a little girl she often saw her mum run. She clearly had inherited her mum's love for movement. It was in those times she connected with herself, her deeper why. It all seemed to come together and make sense.

There are times in life we doubt ourselves.

Maybe we made a wrong turn.

Are we heading the wrong way?

There is a sinking feeling inside of *oooohhh no*.

Someone said something.

It was just a whisper but you heard it anyway.

You could see it on their face.

You question yourself.

You question your own truth.

Then it returns.

As it always does.

That feeling you know.

You are in the right place.

You are in your athletic zone.

Shining and living in your own light.

You notice that familiar feeling.

You sense the excitement inside.

Building.

This is one more step along the road of becoming.

The explorer in you arises.

The deeper knowing inside you arises.

You are in the right place.

This is your moment.
You stand up a little taller.
Shake yourself off.
You stand your ground.
This is your space.
Your truth is strong now.
It sits in your chest, inside your heart.
Your breathing becomes deeper.
You answer your calling.
You lead the way.

AN OLD OAK TREE

Before we step forward into goal setting for your Athlete Within, it is worth taking a moment to visualise yourself moving forward. The big why of your Athlete Within is your why root. When the conditions arise and the storms and chaos of life move in, you are able to stand centred and strong. Every morning, make your why root yours by going back to the feeling of your why. Just like an old oak tree that has seen the test of time, you can imagine yourself as that tree, imagine that the power of the oak's trunk lies in the depth and spread of its root system. It is hard to know someone else's root system, whether it is shallow and easily dislodged when the rain comes, or whether it is a deep why root able to withstand the greatest of storms. The why root is a deep feeling of truth.

Your Athlete Within is bringing out a part of you to the world. Your why is an inside thing that shows up as an external thing. Get it right and you have a life of wonder, greatness and fulfilment.

With this in mind, goal setting becomes an expression of your why root, setting targets and milestones of how you are going to express your why root to the world in the future.

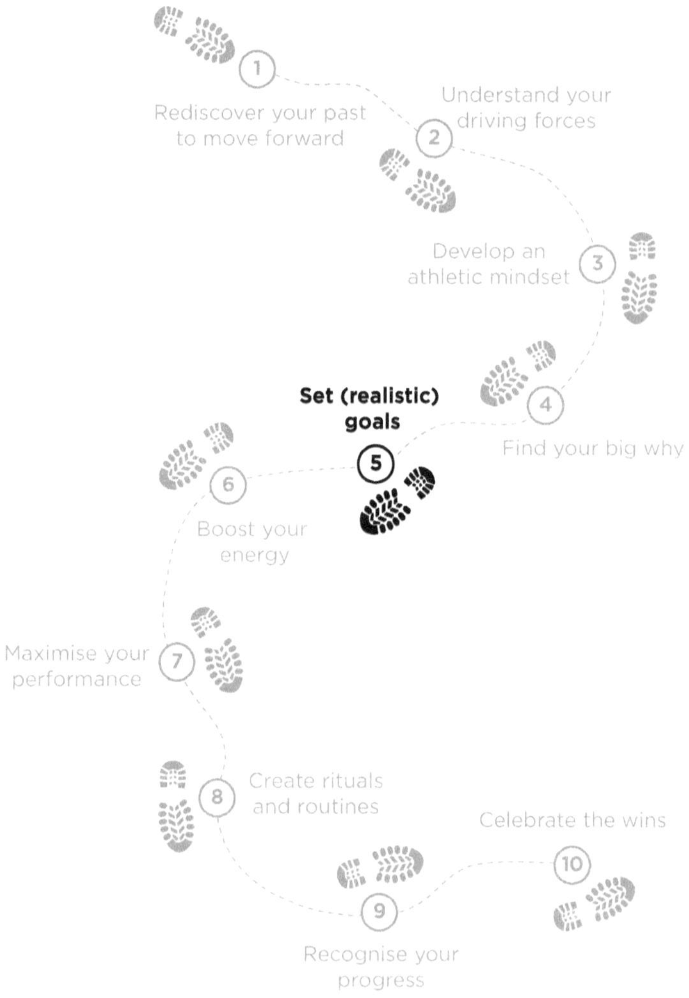

1
Rediscover your past to move forward
2
Understand your driving forces
Develop an athletic mindset
3
4
Find your big why
Set (realistic) goals
5
6
Boost your energy
Maximise your performance
7
Create rituals and routines
8
Celebrate the wins
10
9
Recognise your progress

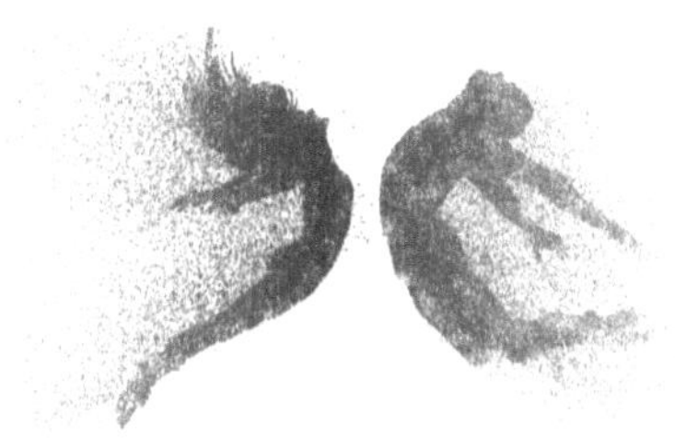

STEP 5:
SET (REALISTIC) GOALS

WHAT YOU WANT THE FUTURE TO BE

Often the words 'goal setting' conjure up a *here we go again* attitude, a reminder of the trail of destruction of previous attempts that failed miserably. Goal setting is really like going on a holiday overseas; there is a map open on the table, you're flicking through scenic pictures from *National Geographic* on your phone, a Lonely Planet book in hand, calling out names of destinations and making a list. As there are already many goal-setting tools and workshops available, in this step I am going to highlight key thoughts to help you define and bring to life your ambitions of your Athlete Within.* The difference is we are working with a framework and this too is part of the process.

---

* The space on goal setting is already so well established that to do it justice would require another volume to this book. There is an incredible number of great resources on goal setting available, such as:

https://www.proctorgallagherinstitute.com/how-to-set-the-right-goals
https://www.tonyrobbins.com/ask-tony/can-create-compelling-future
https://www.jimrohn.com/category/blog/goal-setting

Rediscovering your Athlete Within falls into two phases: the final phase is the destination, reaching the end point of your purpose, knowing you have made it, your Athlete Within. The taste of success and celebration. Yet there is also the first phase, the one that everyone talks about, the one where we make sacrifices, face obstacles, test our abilities, fall down and get back up, learn to become resourceful, learn to become accepting and are humbled, often known as *the journey*.

Goal setting is creating a vision towards your Athlete Within and building the steps to discovering all you can be. Your goals are about bringing your dreams and desires to life, constructing a road map and strategies to move forward, thinking out the possibilities that provide a clearer path on becoming your Athlete Within. Realistic goals are the doing phase. The goals you create are stepping stones you take to your next milestone. As you reach each of your goals, they become vantage points, points where you can look forward and look back, see the learnings, the progress and growth of your Athlete Within.

You are creating a target, in a sense a worthy opponent, striving towards something tangible, something so real you can clearly describe it to another person. Who are you as this athlete? What is it that you love to do? What is it you *can* do?

Realistic goal setting is deciding what you want the future to be, what your ideal Athlete Within looks like, confirmation you are moving in the right direction. Realistic goals begin with your why root. Your why root gives you understanding of the reasons your Athlete Within is important to you, and your goals are about bringing this feeling to life.

Realistic goals are about setting yourself up to win. Goals are destinations you are working towards and each one has a gap you will need to build a bridge across. With time, as you become more confident at goal setting, these bridges may cross greater gaps. Yet a point often missed by many is that goal setting is an art to master in itself. Setting yourself up for success is not about keeping your goals small but keeping them realistic.

It then makes sense there is a process to creating and setting goals so they become shaped and recalibrated along the road. With 'shaping', you move into the nitty gritty of goal setting.

MAKE A PROMISE TO YOURSELF

'Set your eyes on something so big, so exhilarating that it excites you and scares you at the same time.'

Self-help author Bob Proctor

What is your promise of the future? As your Athlete Within, what are your dreams, the things you could be, the way you would like it to be? What do you want to spend more time on? A key to stepping away from the pack and swimming up the river is a clear vision. A vision is what parts the seas.

Let's face it, being active requires effort. It can be exhausting. A vision big enough though will launch you out of the bed and off the couch. It will drive you towards living your best life, being something incredible.

A promise is a declaration that this *will* happen. It is compelling and brings courage. It creates a belief, a story that goes somewhere. The story has to be greater than where you are now, in this moment. We have all made promises to ourselves, promises about who we will be, what we will do in the future, our dreams of what can be. But often we become stuck, lost in the feeling of overwhelm, concerned rather than adventurous, afraid rather than standing with courage.

Conflicting emotions cause distraction and lead to fear and inaction. We just freeze in the moment. Your promise is about stepping into the unknown and not playing small. Knowing your why is your root through the dark times, leaning into the cold southern ice wind towards the light, your destination. All of this requires a keen sense, street smarts, your athletic wisdom to not get caught in the clutter but to find a way forward that opens up and brings freedom. With freedom we have more space for thinking, dreaming and creating more of your Athlete Within.

Exercise

What is your promise of the future? As your Athlete Within, what opportunities and possibilities lie ahead?

Think back to your wishlist. Pick five things, and start with one. Make it big enough it scares you.

GET STARTED

Kylie made a promise. She was travelling through Italy with friends. One night, while enjoying a lovely Italian red, one of her companions made a declaration on his recent retirement. He related a story of how a fellow worker had a heart attack on his third-last day of work, the seed to organising their current trip through the wine regions of Italy. Kylie was so moved by this story, having already set her own retirement plans in place, she started a conversation with her husband that night. You can only imagine how it played out. Thinking about her future plans, she asked her husband why they weren't doing it now – what were they waiting for? He was particularly enjoying this part of his career, could easily take time off, but was not wanting to retire yet. Kylie had more recently purchased a horse and riding lessons, a teenage passion she let go when the kids came along. The PM life in her questioned the want to sit at a desk versus the outdoors on the back of a horse. Her husband said the choice was entirely hers. The second day returning to work she sat down with her boss, who was already smiling. It clearly wasn't a surprise. They planned her retirement there and then. This opened up the door – now she dreamed of more than just riding a horse, she wanted to compete in dressage and she embarked on a new road.

The biggest step in capturing the promise of your future is *starting*. Taking this first step is telling the universe you are serious. As humans we have a unique gift in being able to forward think, plan and deliver. Being realistic is to be serious, to deliver on your own word and demonstrate to the universe that you can.

Exercise

What are your priority constraints?

What is the one thing you have to get past? Often it is living in the past and not directing your promise to the future. Ask yourself if this is the true problem.

What is one thing, one action step, you can do right now?

MAKE YOUR GOALS MEASURABLE

What can you add that can be tangible, easy-to-follow steps to mark where you are on the journey?

Goals are an opportunity to think outside your box. Your wishlist is a list of 'could bes' and 'maybe some days'. Goals are when you pluck one of these ideas out of your wishlist, whisper to yourself *this one* and then you go after it. Now you give it attention, you give it affection, you breathe life into it because of the meaning you give it and connection you make with it. Being specific is adding details about your goal, giving it greater clarity, like it's up on the big screen.

The more detail you can give, the more feeling you bring, the more your brain will focus and look out for anything that takes you closer to your target. It's like building a house; I can take you out to the empty block of land on an imaginary tour, show you where the driveway is, take you up to the front door and through the house. The plans are so real in my head, I know what furniture goes where, which pictures are on the wall and where the dog is lying on the floor, by the window in the sun.

Being specific means having a family of metrics. Humans love numbers to discuss and compare but there is meaning in the data – analysis gives insight. Without detail and a clear understanding of your path forward, you can quickly fall into overwhelm and clutter. Don't confuse the feeling of busy with progress. The noise of the environment clogs up our filter, pulling us off track. Specifics keep us sharp with deliberate attention, coming back to why we are doing this, the feeling of living in the moment. It is the specifics that keep you out of the pull of distraction.

For the Athlete Within, metrics are a working model, a way to know where you are at and when you are moving forwards towards your targets. Keeping it relevant, not clinical, means staying in touch with the feeling of your goals, not getting lost in the numbers. Gauging your energy levels, ticking off your emotional level of engagement, your feeling of where you are at shows up patterns of how connected you are to your realistic goals. You may choose wearable technology to measure a family of metrics like VO2, HRV, HR and other factors, but keep asking yourself, is this going to help me towards my athletic pursuit? Is this going to give me stepping stones I can use to create momentum?

Often we create our goals without properly paying attention to time. We have inherent expectations that if not properly thought out quickly pull us away from our desired intention. Time is about pacing yourself, paying attention to where you are in the moment, being present. Do not be fooled by the foul play of time, it is lurking and toying, testing your truth and desire to meet your goals. Remember that time is a human invention in our world looking to control, whereas becoming lost in time is being absorbed in your own path to truth.

Goals are a way forward, it is leadership from the inside. It is planting your flag in the ground. Being specific means being clear. The flipside of this is to be able to measure it – there are tangible targets and markers along the way to navigate by. In some ways it isn't about hitting every marker or being there at the designated time – it is about the pursuit of your promise.

A place to start is to consider all the obstacles and challenges that have stopped you in the past and then flip them 180 degrees and see where they land. This is facing the challenge, being clear about the problem and then, as Professor Stuart McGill so aptly describes, 'playing jazz'. Change it, see it differently, make it exciting, dress it up in a way that causes an explosion.

Exercise

Being specific is to bring clarity to your goal. Describe the moment, the exact time in the future when you know you have arrived:

- Where are you?

- Who is with you?

- What are you looking at?

- What was the story leading up to this moment?

- What was the crunch, the biggest obstacle?

- How does it feel to be here, to have arrived?

- And what is your next goal?

Just thinking about these questions already brings you up to the starting line.

MAKE YOUR GOALS MEANINGFUL

'This life is more than just a read-through.'

Red Hot Chilli Peppers

Your goals need to be meaningful. When you are working on you, the effort is reward. You are ticking your boxes, you are spending time in your three spheres.

Jim Rohn talks about the promise of the future, understanding that the journey will go through cycles, its seasons. Winter is for getting ready, the preparation for spring's crops and moving forward into the summer harvest. The farmer begins with a clear vision, a story we all know well. Of course the seasons change, some crops succeed, some fail, but the farmer keeps showing up year after year, building the dream and providing for the family.

It was self-help author Bob Proctor who gave insight on this path. Your big why has meaning, it holds greatness, it is the root that keeps you strongly anchored to your Athlete Within. Set a promise of the future that meets the Proctor criteria: if it doesn't scare you, it ain't big enough. When you feel something so strong you just can't contain it anymore, you have to take action. Your true promise requires boldness and faith. Of course there are other roads, easier roads, yet they don't have the same feeling, the same meaning, the same promise, the chance to explore your greatness.

Personally, I have danced often with this step, playing a small game and feeling great at it, preferring comfort to standing up. Cancer changed my viewpoint. It gave me the insight of bigness and changed how high I set my bar. I learnt it was about embracing the fear and doing it anyway. It's not that I throw myself into high-intensity situations, I more 'slow burn it'. I do it incrementally. Even turning it up from the previous chapter, being more deliberate about my rehearsal, working in situations that make it more real. If it is an athletic event for example, I will actually go to the location, probably early on a Sunday morning, walk the course, take photos of key sections, make a video where I'm crossing the finish line. All this making it more familiar, closer and more real, ready for the actual event itself.

BE OPEN MINDED

'The big challenge is to become all that you have the possibility of becoming. You cannot believe what it does to the human spirit to maximise your human potential and stretch yourself to the limit.'

Jim Rohn

As we move forward towards our realistic goals rediscovering our Athlete Within, we want to keep an open mind, not become lost in our rules, but be able to flex, absorb the falls and bounce.

To design our realistic goals to bring them to life, make them more real, follow the principles, you want to work on making them specific, include enough details where someone else could follow through on your action steps. They are meaningful, they connect you to your why root, engage you, excite you, they compel you to keep moving forward and they are achievable. Each goal is just a step to a new vantage point. They allow you to back your life story, the lessons you have onboarded, and see further forward to who you are becoming.

So it only makes sense now to move our attention to energy, because you need a bucketload of it to bring on change.

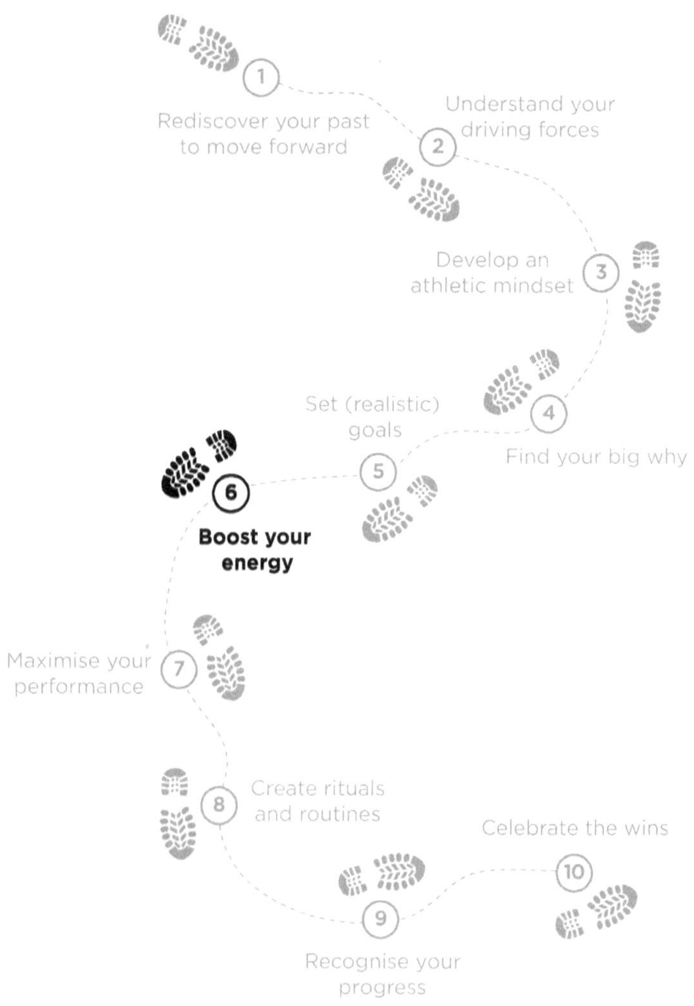

1
Rediscover your past to move forward
2
Understand your driving forces
3
Develop an athletic mindset
4
Find your big why
5
Set (realistic) goals
6
Boost your energy
7
Maximise your performance
8
Create rituals and routines
9
Recognise your progress
10
Celebrate the wins

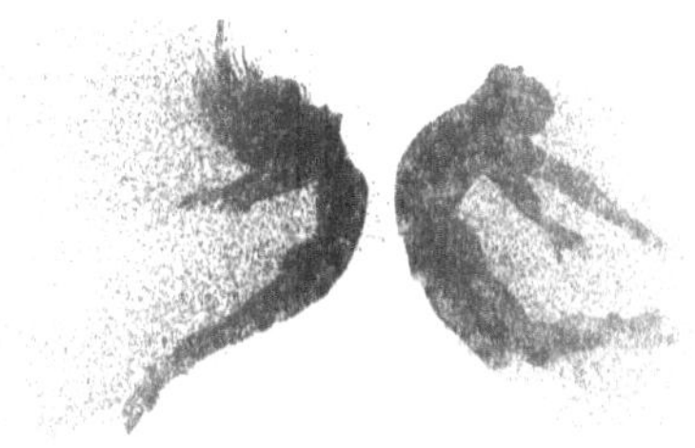

STEP 6:
BOOST YOUR ENERGY

WHAT IS ENERGY AND WHY DO YOU NEED IT?

How do you know you have energy? Well, it's more of a feeling than something we can put our hands on. We know when we wake up in the morning whether we're ready to get up and seize the day or whether we can't even be bothered getting out of bed. Having energy is being ready for anything. A big day at work, a weekend away, a beach outing with the kids that we are actually looking forward to. For your Athlete Within it also means you're ready for change.

So how do we get more energy? One approach is to look at food. What we eat will affect our system and play with our energy. But food is only one element of what influences our level of energy – that's not the full picture. Most of us are trained to think about energy like a switch you can flick on by simply addressing one thing. You swallow this, eat that, remove a few things that may cause resistance and the body can feel energy magically take place. This armchair approach is often linear and one dimensional, and although simplicity can often be a good thing, our biology is much greater than the sum of the parts; we are multidimensional beings. So we need to go deeper and look at other aspects of our body and lifestyle to have a long-lasting effect on our energy levels.

For a moment, I want you to think of your body's energy as a system controlled by five dials on a dashboard, and each of these dials can be turned up or down depending on external and internal factors. Food is only one of these dials; the others are dials you might be familiar with but you might not necessarily have paid much attention to (so far):

- breathing
- sleeping
- timing (your internal rhythm)
- movement.

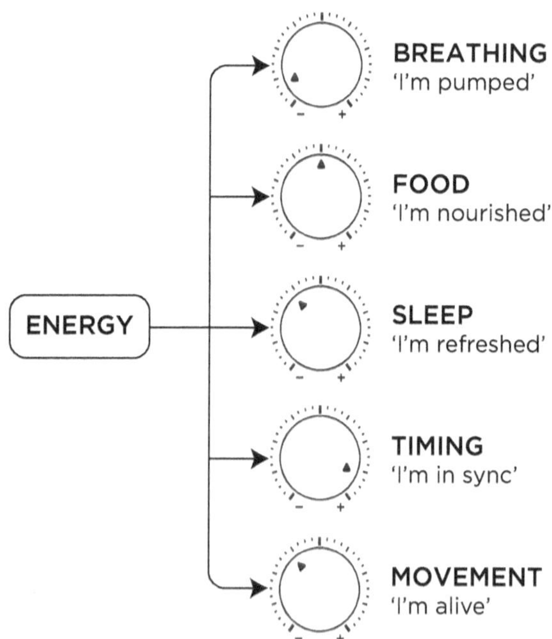

When you look at one of these dials and tune it, you might find an instant change in your energy. It's like drinking a shot of coffee mid-afternoon to give you a burst to get you to the end of the day. But if you do this you are starting the yo-yo cycle, and for every higher up there is a lower down. Even though some dials may be more significant to you, you have to remember that every dial – if compromised at some level – leaves you with a deficiency which can lead you all the way down the road of chronicity: the big scary health conditions.

The aim of your Athlete Within is to understand, manage and tune all the dials the way that is just right for you, for your individual dashboard, so you can increase your energy level day in day out, without pushing the system to exhaustion. It's about building longevity and sustainability.

Lack of energy is something we all experience at some point in our lives, and even though we are living in an era of greater life expectancy, the way we are enjoying it is less enthusiastic, dragging around fatigue that can easily turn into illnesses. Remember the stats? By the time we reach 70 years, eight out of ten of us will carry two or more chronic illnesses, hitched on like an unwanted heavy backpack.

One of my close friends, Chris, is at that time in his life when he is unfortunately moving through a divorce. He is at that point, you know where you start to lift your head up, look around and realise there is still a world outside. Wanting to get healthier again and get back to reality, he decided to join a gym and asked me for some advice. Together, we quickly realised he needed to do more than just focus on the gym:

- His life was a day-to-day adventure story, so slowing things down and adding some organisation was a key for this to be a lasting episode. We started with going to bed 40 minutes earlier every night. He had this habit of staying up, turning on some kind of device or watching the end of something. Then the cascade took over: he was up a little later, felt a little hungrier, began snacking a little more, the weight started to grow, he was more tired getting out of bed.

- At the gym, rather than hitting it hard, it was about finding a rhythm. He liked the idea of boxing classes. They are social and interactive. He started a weight program and thought about some tennis.

- The key here was slow entry. He was out of condition, but he wasn't training for a Hollywood role or a competition, so he could set the pace at 'slow burn' (something I base my whole thinking on and it's coming to you in its full glory in Step 7). He could set a realistic timeframe and expectations that were compelling and achievable.

- Then we considered the recovery factor. He had been on the divorce roller-coaster for a while and working full time. His head was in many places, none of which were calm. We also discussed slow bike sessions, just spinning and turning over the wheels, or floating in the pool like a kid and spending time in the spa. Letting himself go, letting his mind wander and to just be. This was the hardest part. It felt to him like a waste of time with no real purpose, but finding and training his Athlete Within wasn't just a physical experience. He needed to re-find his enjoyment, his own meaning and purpose, and think out some of his future steps and dreams.

This all fell into three short steps, the hardest he admitted was beginning the sleep time routine and shifting some of his habits, making the bedroom his sanctuary for sleep. Chris was out of tune. He needed to look at his individual dashboard and work out where his dials should be.

To become your Athlete Within you are going to have to make some changes, make new choices, take a leap, face some conflict, move through a period of being uncomfortable along the road to becoming.

To do this, you need fire in the belly – you need energy. In a crazy twist, it's like needing energy to make changes to increase energy.

Changing your internal and external environments is very powerful. It's taking out all the parts that aren't really you, the triggers that cause you frustration or rob you of your energy, so you can find your own clarity and reinforce your proximity. What are you carrying around with you in your heavy backpack that letting go of would energise you and give you freedom to rediscover your Athlete Within?

Let's get started.

DIAL 1: HOW TO GET YOUR BREATHING RIGHT

Breathing is such an underrated affair. It just happens. We don't really think about it and we certainly don't put much attention to it because we do it so many times during the day (and night). It is just another function that keeps us alive.

However, breathing efficiently may not be as easy as you think. In our world made out of sedentary habits and ruled by deconditioning, regaining our ability to breathe properly requires a bit of focus, just as you would when building muscles. Breathing becomes a skill that requires time to develop and coordination to master. Breathing is trainable.

Before Chris decided to work on his Athlete Within, he was overweight, overtired and overwhelmed. The endless hours spent sitting at his desk and the lack of activity meant his body was not in great shape, he was fatiguing easily and ran out of breath very quickly. Blowing up a balloon for his kid's birthday party gave him head spins, and walking up the stairs left him breathless. At night it was more of the same. He was snoring, he was restless, and was waking up more and more tired each day.

When we think of breathless Chris trying to climb a flight of stairs or restless Chris having an apnoea episode in his sleep, we imagine him gasping for air, unable to draw enough oxygen in. But the truth is, the oxygen levels in the body of a healthy adult don't fluctuate.

To form the full picture we also need to look at how we exhale. Breathing out is an important function to dispose of carbon dioxide (the exhaust from burning oxygen) as well as the waste products from our metabolism. The diaphragm is the primary muscle driving the way we breathe, pushing down like a piston, it draws air in and expands our rib cage. It is also responsible for influencing spinal stabilisation and the way we control movement in our bodies. Because of our lifestyles, our breathing has moved more into our upper chest directly affecting the tension around our necks and the way we exhale from our lungs. As a result, we can often experience neck stiffness, back pain, headaches, and cannot dispose efficiently of all our metabolic waste.

Because Chris is not in the greatest form of his life (yet), his breathing is small, fast and shallow, when ideally he should be taking full advantage of his diaphragm and drawing fewer breaths, slowing the process down and exhaling more deeply. He has forgotten he has a lovely nose that can help him take in fresh air and optimise his breathing, instead he uses his big (loud) mouth. His shallow breathing pattern makes for an increased level of carbon dioxide in his system, bringing on the urge to blow out more and become breathless. At night, when the back of his mouth and tongue collapse, blocking his airways, his brain is able to detect the build up of poisonous carbon dioxide and jolt the body awake to take a breath.

Human beings are masters of endurance: we are 16 times more efficient when we breathe enough oxygen to meet our needs and fuel our activities. What it means for your Athlete Within is that, ideally, you need to strive to achieve aerobic respiration, that sweet spot when you're using your body at its capacity and you can still have a nice chat about life. Why? Because when you talk you need to breathe out to make sounds in sync with your exercise. Also, it's way more fun.

To achieve aerobic respiration is to tune your breathing dial to its optimum level, yet few of us are aware of how to train the diaphragm and our breathing. Let's start by taking a look at your breathing first. The following thoughts and ideas will help you paint a picture of how you are breathing and offer some suggestions on how to improve the way you breathe:

- **Are you a mouth breather?** Your nose plays an important role. It is your immune system's detection inspector and prepares outside air for your inside, warming it up and filtering out the nasties. Mouth breathing bypasses all these essential activities. Do you wake up in the morning with a dry mouth, bad breath and feeling tired? Does your nose become easily blocked or itchy? Do you snore? These can be signs of mouth breathing and even sleep apnoea.

- **Can you exhale well and slowly?** Your ability to exhale can have a ripple effect on other areas of your body: when you increase your lung capacity and slow your breath, you shift your neurology, you are pulled into parasympathetic mode (decreasing your stress response and racing thoughts) and improving your ability to blow out carbon dioxide. James Nestor in his book *Breath* takes you into this world in greater detail as well as outlining techniques to improve your breathing.

- **Use your breathing as a powerful metric.** If you are walking or running or climbing a hill, are you able to keep breathing through your nose? Are you able to hold a conversation? This way you're keeping within aerobic respiration, driving your energy levels and not exhausting the system.

Once you know if you're breathing at your optimal level, you can start training your breath and work on your diaphragm just like any other muscle in your body. Consistency and deliberate intention are key. I suggest starting small and integrating breathing into your rituals and routines:

- **Train your aerobic respiration.** Go for a 20-minute walk. Aim to keep your lips sealed through the whole journey. To start with, take note of the moment this may become difficult. Second, increase your pace to your top range, where you reach a point you want to switch to mouth breathing (but don't go there!). Third, keep the pace and concentrate on your exhaling and expelling carbon dioxide. Lastly, drop back a gear and find a pace, your pace, that you can keep while staying in aerobic respiration.

- **Train your diaphragm.** There is one exercise I absolutely love and I teach it to all my clients. It is simple, it doesn't require any equipment and can be done at any time of the day, wherever you are. To me it is the one exercise every Athlete Within should master. You can find it here: **www.brettlillie.com/ breathingexercise**

- **Give meditation a go.** Meditation is breathing in mindfulness. Meditation can be guided following a visual journey, or it may simply centre around awareness of your breath. Mediation can be sitting quietly and going in, or heading outside for a walk along the beach and spending time in nature. It is time for solitude, silence and reflection. It is time with you and your rhythm, your breath.

Exercise

Integrate breathing activities into your morning routine to prime yourself, ready for the day. Concentrate on developing one aspect of your breathing. Inhale. Exhale. Slow. Hold the space when you breathe out.

Add a movement – stretch and breath through it.

DIAL 2: HOW TO GET YOUR FOOD RIGHT

'Kids that grow kale, eat kale.'

The Gangster Gardener

When I was diagnosed with cancer at 44, I was in shock and disbelief, but I knew I wasn't ready to go just yet. The surgery removed 26 cm of colon; as a friend put it, had it been outside my body I would have lost half of my arm.

Out of the hospital and into the bookstore, I wanted to start reading and educating myself on food in relation to my health, but oh the confusion; carb vs no carb; protein rich or raw; eat for diabetes; eat for menopause (not quite for me); detox; coloured diets; farm to table. Plus books on food technology, food industry, food allergies, food pyramids, food everything. On TV we had just shelved *The Biggest Loser* and replaced it with *MasterChef*, a show on how to enjoy food. More confusion. So I took a step back and started reading about paleo and Mediterranean diets.

The truth is we run on ancient algorithms and food habits: strategies that worked for our ancestors. Enter the paleo concept, a thinking that speaks to the scientist in me and has had a deep influence in how I approach food. It is the idea that we evolved to eat the same way our hunter and gatherer relatives did in the paleolithic days. Even with the arrival of the agricultural era, our genes haven't quite had the chance to truly catch up and adapt to farmed foods or the soft, refined, processed diets of today.

Cancer taught me many lessons, and with such new knowledge I decided to take my nutrition very seriously, targeting a diet high in raw food, good oils, nuts and seeds with only high-quality meat. Surgery had reduced my available real estate for my biome to inhabit, so I knew I had to nurture whatever was left and introduced pre- and probiotic foods, including superfoods and fermented foods: blueberries, kale, beans, yogurts, kimchi, sauerkraut and the like.

For me, what I ate and the way I ate were a key part of my cancer story. Raw food meant I had to chew more, initiating digestion right in my mouth. I was watching how much space I left between meals and snacks. I was connecting to my food and the food source, picking tomatoes off the plants in my backyard, harvesting zucchini and salad. I made a point of truly enjoying my meals and sat at the table with my family and friends, something my wife learnt when she was little growing up in the Italian part of Switzerland where food was fresh and meant to be shared.

My five-year cancer check up was a chance for me to revisit my approach, so I ventured deeper into the research. I discovered that, after all, we don't exactly know what our palaeolithic ancestors ate as it is very difficult to follow the evidence through archaeology. The conclusion: we are simply opportunistic omnivores, we grab whatever we can find. No wonder we'd rather pack our trolleys with ready meals than growing our food. It's convenient, it fits with our routines, we take the opportunity and run.

Shifting your approach to food

Eating packaged food was all Aaron could master. One day, in the clinic, he opened up and confessed he was feeling upset about the weight he was piling on. He was jumping between diets, at first succeeding, losing the kilos but then putting them back on ... and more. I knew we had to shift our conversation from diet to food roots. We talked about his upbringing (rediscovery is so powerful, isn't it?), his face lighting up as he described the wonders of Greek food his grandma laid out on the tables. You could see him coming into his Athlete Within. He ran home, made a Greek salad, yaya's style, and began his journey back to his roots. The weight stayed off, the smile turned up.

In his book *The Hungry Brain*, Stephan Guyenet sheds some light on how our brains are wired up to the sensory input to food. Our 9-to-5 schedule has contributed to the timing for breakfast, lunch and dinner but also those morning and afternoon gaps where we tend to snack right at the point we are most tired, stressed or overworked. Our brain now knows when we need to eat, when we are full, but also what we are nutritionally attracted to – all wired up to a crazy reward system. We want more fats, more sugar – and then we're left hungry for more.

Shifting your approach to food and the ideas you have around eating can be complex and often has a lot of emotional connotations attached to it. Having a good relationship with food is an aim of your inner athlete. You've heard it all before: anything in moderation, just like the French do. Allow yourself to explore with food, knowing what's preferred and what's a treat, remembering that if you eat cake today you don't have to train harder tomorrow – just keep doing you, be active, be your Athlete Within.

Fear not, this is not another diet book. I just want to help you tweak your food energy dial so you can feel nourished and satisfied, and you can think of food as an amazing fuel that can give you joy and send your taste buds flying. So here are some recommendations to start exploring options and see what works for you:

- Start with research guidelines. I would personally head towards a combination of paleo and Mediterranean diets. At the end of the day, as Professor Herman Pontzer puts it, every diet works as long as you stick to it. And if consistency and willpower are not your best friends, remember that your Athlete Within can work on these by checking in on your mindset (see Step 3). Make your approach to food meaningful, make it yours, make it fun, give it a big why and you'll give yourself an amazing base to start your journey.

- Just as you went back to rediscover your inner athlete, go back and check in on your dietary roots. What did your parents and grandparents eat? What variety of food did they cook and prepare? Are you still incorporating these foods into your daily intake? If not, when and why did you stop? What was your childhood preferred dish? Does your family have a secret recipe that your grandmother has passed down?

- Take a moment to look at what you eat on a daily basis. How's your nutritional profile? A good point to start from is to eat a bit of everything in moderation, but focus on eating raw and whole foods. Avoid packaged food (or at least the labels with more than five ingredients). Does it contain fat or sugar? Often low fat means high sugar. Eat what's in season (plenty of fibre – your biome's favourite food) and, even better, eat local produce so you know you're getting the most nutrients. Maybe explore your local farmers' market.

- When it comes to veggies, load up to help slow down your digestion. This keeps you feeling full for longer and gives you great fuel.

- If you eat highly refined food such as sugar, your digestion speeds up, making you want to eat again. (Have you noticed how you're often hungry after a big McDonald's meal? That's why.) Also, the refining process removes a lot of nutrients, minerals and even fibre. Sometimes such meals are referred to as 'empty calories'.

- Do you like gardening? Maybe it's time to start growing some food, even just starting with a pot of herbs. This will give you a chance to reconnect with nature and with the produce you put on your plate. Nothing is quite as satisfying as picking your own food and eating it right away, still warm from the sun.

- Chew more. Your digestion starts in your mouth. When you chew you start to break down food, making it easier for your body to absorb nutrients. Plus, you're keeping your biting and facial equipment in top shape.

- Remember to hydrate. Often we feel hungry when in reality we're just thirsty.

- Snacking is perfectly okay. If you're hungry your body needs food. Have some water first and if you're still hungry after 20 minutes, tuck in. If you tend to grab whatever is easily available (usually what comes in a pack in the pantry), here are some things you can do to help you make great snack choices:

  - Prepare food: cut up some veggies so they're ready when you're hungry. I love a good trail mix, and that's another easy thing to do.
  - Graze: you don't have to eat three square meals a day. If you prefer to eat at shorter intervals, do that and adjust your portion sizes.
  - Reconsider your proximity – what food is within easy reach?

- If snacking is your late-night enemy, I'd suggest you go to bed earlier but I know I'd be banging on the wrong door. Maybe brush your teeth after dinner – who on earth would bother brushing their teeth twice (I want to hear from you if you do), plus ice-cream *never* tastes good after mint toothpaste.

- Check the size of your portions and the overall amount of your food intake. This is particularly important if you're trying to shift weight. Start by balancing your energy expenditure equation: if you eat more than you burn, you gain weight. If you eat too little you go into starvation mode and your brain will be triggered to store fat. Here's the catch – we all tend to burn the same amount of calories each day, whether you are The Rock training for the next movie or you're sitting at your desk for 12 hours in your office.

· What gives you more energy is the way your body responds to exercise (an active lifestyle is key), assisted by eating quality, nutritious food efficiently, and not the quantity of food you eat. When you are talking about weight, decreasing calorie intake is your first step. Physical activity on its own doesn't change the number of calories we burn, but it does change the way we spend those calories. Fill up on low-carb, high-fibre veggies to decrease calorie intake.

· When do you tend to eat? Research shows that we shouldn't go near food just before we go to bed, yet the evenings are often a stomping ground for snackers. When you eat is as important as what you eat. Nighttime fasting (for 8 to 12 hours) ensures that you're not digesting when you are going to bed so your brain can truly concentrate on carrying out its night functions (growing, processing, consolidating, cleaning, regenerating).

· What about planning ahead? I know this could feel a bit like another item to add to your long to-do list, but planning gets rid of the 'what's for dinner' stress many of us feel when we get home from work late in the evening and we open the fridge hoping for meal inspiration, and it saves money too. Another little trick is to cook double the amount you need for dinner so lunchboxes become super easy to fill the following day: grab leftovers, and add veggies, one piece of fruit and a mid-morning snack.

Even just incorporating *one* of these recommendations can have a huge impact on your energy level. My last thought: make incremental changes – eating is habitual. Time is on your side. Small tweaks allow for your system to adjust, absorb and get ready for the next step.

Exercise

What is the one thing you have learnt that you can implement right away to create good food habits that nourish? Remember the answer to what works for you could lie in your past - make it your own.

DIAL 3: HOW TO GET YOUR SLEEP RIGHT

'An hour of sleep before midnight is worth two after.'

Confucius

Oh we do love our sleep, don't we? Ask a new parent what is the thing they're missing the most and the answer will most probably be sleep. That feeling of waking up in the morning ready to tackle anything after an uninterrupted night in the land of nod. But when was the last time *you* woke up feeling refreshed? In my clinic this is one of my favourite questions. Often there is no quick answer. Lost in thought, trying to remember, people just seem to glaze over, unsure of a time. That is a telling sign the sleep dial has been neglected for a while.

Sleep is a crucial window into your lifestyle, a dial to measure how your body and you are coping, and is a major contributor to energy levels. Reaching optimum sleep means you're able to fall asleep easily and stay asleep throughout the night, making the most of the dark and all that your sleep cycles can offer. Good sleep is not about shutting *down* but rather shutting *out* the world and letting your brain change gears.

Yet, we are constantly faced with crazy pressures and expectations about how much more we can squeeze into each day: more deadlines, more work, more emails that require a reply at any time of the day or night, more late Zoom meetings. Wasn't it Margaret Thatcher who said 'sleep is for wimps'? And so we soldier on, like the Iron Lady. If we look around, people seem to achieve so much, leaving us questioning our own commitment, our own value in the world, so we put sleep further down the priority list and coffee up. In fact, we sleep on average two hours less than our grandparents did.

It's no surprise sleep is such a big topic right now. There are so many apps and products to try to help people fall asleep and have a good night's rest. Even though many influential names in the executive world – the likes of Jeff Bezos – are starting to beat the drum of the 'you need eight hours of sleep' to operate at your best, it's fair to say that among the population sleep has declined along with physical activity.

A lot of us seem to survive on six hours of sleep, but when you start to read the fine print, the stats are pretty dreadful. So many aspects of our lives can be affected by lack of sleep. Compromised sleep can lead to chronic stress and chronic pain. Sleep deficiency decreases alertness, so we have to learn to adapt and resort to external aids such as coffee and sugar to help our bodies stay awake and cope with the demands of daily life (hello bigger waistline). Less sleep or, better put, decreased sleep quality leads to a drop in energy and motivation. It decreases our life expectancy. It pushes inflammation up and increases neurotoxins so our body can't clean out the nasties or heal properly. Lack of sleep stresses our cardiovascular system and puts a load on our metabolic system leading to weight gain, insulin resistance, diabetes and even cancer. On top of that, when we don't sleep enough we become clumsy, we make mistakes, we fall asleep at the wheel. And the emotional load associated with poor sleep means moodiness, increased anxiety, depression and risk of suicide. Pretty grim.

When rediscovering your Athlete Within, lack of sleep can affect performance and pull energy away from motivation, mindset and clarity. We carry the pressure of sleep through the day, feeling so tired and bored we want to nod off, to then reach bedtime and we are wide awake, wondering, thinking, not able to fall asleep.

Time to park the negative stuff, get down to business and go over some great strategies we can use to improve the quality of our sleep and turn up the dial to our optimum level. Actually, maybe now is a great time to get out of your chair for a few minutes (or bed if you're reading lying down) and pick up the book again after a good stretch. Or even better, get out for a quick walk around the block. You'll sleep better tonight for it.

To manage our sleep dial we need to gain some understanding of what happens when we are asleep, how sleep works and what we can do to make it our best friend.

First of all, it's important to know that when we go to sleep our brain does not shut off, done, closed for business, goodnight, rather it becomes very active and performs functions that are vital to gaining optimal energy we can then use during the day. Even though for a long time darkness and sleep were seen as wasted downtime, we now understand that at night the brain is able to cut off sensory information from the outside world to change gears and get to work, processing all the information acquired during the day. Sleep is not about rest, it's about reset.

Each night sleep is made up of many different cycles that each last about 90 minutes. Each cycle can be broken down into two parts, referred to as deep slow-wave sleep (SWS) or delta sleep, and rapid eye movement (REM) sleep. These two stages are in constant battle for domination of the brain's attention (they just want to be picked), and they fight in what Professor Matthew Walker refers to as the Cerebral War. Each war is won and lost every sleep cycle and then it repeats. In the earlier stages of the night it is your deep SWS that tends to dominate the battle, but as the night rolls on it is your REM sleep that takes centre stage, bringing sleep home to morning.

As we close our eyes, most of us drift into sleep within about 20 minutes, stepping down the stairs into the chambers of deep slow-wave sleep. At this point all the muscles in your body are deactivated, except your diaphragm and some eye muscles. Your metabolism is slowing down to about 10% to 15%, your temperature drops, your brain's electrical activity changes. As the brain is super busy during the day learning, processing and managing everything you think and do, it's only during this sleep phase that it can let its many millions of neurons sync and dance together, transferring, consolidating and storing information (did you know we actually do 80% of our growth at night?). It's also in this phase that we can clean our system of all the neurotoxins – the waste from our brain cells – accumulated during the day. Without this flushing mechanism, these sticky neurotoxins tend to aggregate, clogging up the system, killing off neurons and causing plaques we currently associate with Alzheimer's.

It's in the REM phase that we do most of our dreaming, actively acting out our thoughts. Thank goodness our muscle system is disconnected in this phase or whoever is sleeping next to you may cop the brunt of your acting out. We are in a state similar to when we are awake and alert; our vitals are up, including blood pressure, heart rate and even breathing. There is a lot of processing of emotional content, remembering thoughts and memories, cutting and pruning, consolidating strong emotional content and clearing out our memory sticks preparing us for the new day ahead. This is particularly important in things like studying for an exam. Turns out the brain needs to clear out what's on the mental desk (thoughts and emotions) before onloading new info as well as processing and consolidating.

Research gives us guidelines to work with. Best current knowledge recommends we get eight hours of sleep per night. This allows for the appropriate amount of SWS and REM sleep to take place, letting the cerebral war pan out naturally, with both contenders winning and losing at the right time of the sleep cycle.

So what happens if you cut sleep short? Most of your REM sleep happens in the last two hours at the end of the night, so if you give yourself six hours sleep, you are only cutting your sleep time down by

25% but you are actually decreasing your REM sleep by a staggering 70%. The results can be seen when you wake up: foggy mind, mood swings, lack of energy and motivation, unbalanced hormone levels, you are more sensitive to pain and may feel quite anxious.

A major contributor to poor sleep habits is actually us – yes, you and me – with our annoying aversion to a bedtime routine and ritual, because really, only kids have a bath, read a book and then go to sleep at the same time every night. Other disruptive factors are allergies, high consumption of coffee and alcohol, airway issues, stress and lack of movement during the day.

Everyone has their own dashboards to generate energy, and the sleep dial, just like the others, is very individual. There is no single pattern for sleep. Some of us are heavy sleepers, others wake at the slightest noise. Some have the tendency to go to bed early (me), others (my wife) are night owls who thrive after 10 pm. Being in tune with our body means knowing what we need to address and what changes we might want to introduce to improve our sleep quality.

Sleep is about looking for underlying patterns rather than treating the symptoms. In light of this, I am going to give you some suggestions to help you understand your own sleep pattern and offer ideas on what to do to minimise disruptive sleep and maximise your energy. These are guidelines and what you choose to address needs to work for you. To achieve optimal sleep hygiene, I recommend starting slow but keeping it up. Consistency is key.

- Let's start by looking at your sleep environment. What we surround ourselves with and how we use the space we live in can have a huge impact on our wellbeing. Your bedroom is no different. Let's go through some ideas to ensure the room you sleep in is set up in a way that is conducive to falling asleep and staying asleep:

- Your bedroom is for sleep (and mating). Make it your happy place where you can slow down, take a breath, relax and enjoy.
- Keep it tidy. Exterminate any pile that finds its way into your space, whether this be books, clothes or other stuff.
- Block out the light; use curtains.
- Consider the inside light too – don't rely on the main switch, make sure you have super soft light at your disposal near your bed (fairy lights, warm globes in bedside table lamps, salt rock lamps).
- Set rules and boundaries on what is allowed and not allowed in your bedroom environment. My first suggestion is always to outlaw phones and TVs due to them being so easily accessible with their bright light, noise and distraction.
- Make your bedroom inviting. Decorate it, add candles, nice music and deck it out. Take pride in your room and make your bed every morning.
- Make your room comfortable. Make sure you are sleeping on a good mattress (that you love) and a pillow that supports you. This is very personal and very important.
- Finally, it should be a place of solitude, silence and stillness. Take out the arguments, the food and work – they do not belong in your sanctuary.

· Let's look deeper into your environment to get rid of potential allergens and irritants:

- Consider your room's air environment such as temperature, breeding ground for nasties or moisture traps.
- Open your bedroom up as much as you can to direct sun and breeze.
- Keep it clean – vacuum and dust regularly.

- Machine wash all bed linen at least every two weeks at above 55 degrees Celsius. Hang your covers out in the sun.
- Invest in a mattress cover that protects against dust mites and other nasties.
- Keep a tidy room. Things left around attract moisture and dust and block airflow.

- Look at your sleep routine. A sleep routine is fundamental for the Athlete Within as sleep is about priming, not switching off, and it requires some preparation. So here are some ideas you can grab to incorporate into your own rituals and routine:
  - Create a realistic routine. If you feel at your best in the evening, don't try to go to bed at 9 pm or it'll just go against your grain. You may want to start your bedtime routine at around that time so you feel at your greatest when you're getting ready to go to sleep and you can inject more pleasure into the whole process and give it more meaning.
  - Exercise during the day as it will benefit every facet of your sleep. Avoid moderate to high-intensity exercise two to three hours before sleep, particularly as it raises your core body temperature.
  - Have a good nap, but not later than mid-afternoon. If you're feeling tired during the day or need emotional first aid, either nap for 20 minutes (and wake before you enter deep sleep) or allow 60 to 90 minutes so you don't wake up mid sleep cycle.
  - Steer off caffeine and alcohol in the later part of the day: your body takes six to eight hours to break this stuff down.
  - Eat light, chew a lot, and finish eating two to three hours before sleep time.
  - Start your routine two to three hours before you go to sleep so you can really change gears and transition from daytime

to nighttime. Make the last hour light – I recommend a good book. As we are creatures of habit it is important to develop a daily system that works on the weekend too.

Exercise

Ask yourself these questions and maybe use some of the answers to measure your progress. You may want to journal your thoughts as they can become stepping stones towards your very own individual sleep ritual and preferences:

- When was the last time you woke feeling refreshed? Did you bounce? Or did you feel blah, maybe even run down, or do you not even bother trying to feel energised?
- Do you get to sleep easily? Do you stay asleep or wake during the night?
- Do you experience tiredness during the day? If you lay down, could you close your eyes and drift off to sleep right now?
- Is your bedroom environment conducive to sleep?
- Do you follow a sleep hygiene ritual (schedule and plan)? Is there conflict or stress around your sleep routine?
- Consider your mental and cognitive health. Do you make time for you? Do you use breathing strategies or meditation?
- Does physical exercise and recovery form part of your sleep hygiene?

DIAL 4: HOW TO GET YOUR TIMING RIGHT

Every year you and 60 billion people across 71 countries participate in the largest research project on the planet: daylight saving. We only shift the clocks by a tiny hour to align with our changing external environment: surely this is not a problem at all. Well, the data emerging from such an insignificant shift (in the grand scheme of things) is staggering. Just by losing an hour of sleep when the time changes people increase their risk of heart attack by 24%. And what about jetlag? When we travel far and wide, it takes our bodies 24 hours to absorb a one-hour time difference to get back in sync. You do the maths. Social jetlag is no different: if you wake up every morning at 6 am to go to work and then you sleep in at the weekend, you are messing around with your timing dial.

Now picture yourself taking part in another fun project. Imagine moving deep underground into a cave for 40 days and 40 nights in the name of research. You won't be seeing the light of day. You won't have a clock, your phone, your socials, any news, contact with family or friends, or anything to do with the outside world. Sound enticing? The last time this kind of research was conducted was in 2021 in France, where a group of 15 people went underground to live as they would normally above ground.

In this cave they lived in tents and generated their own electricity by pedalling on bikes. Researchers monitored everything possible: their blood and hormone levels, cognitive function, body temperature, food going in, digestion and biome with a camera swallowed as a pill, then fluid and the like coming out, social behaviours, activity levels, when they went to sleep, what time they woke up and whatever else they could track.

The results? Amazingly, most of the participants enjoyed the experience, didn't realise how long they were down there for and, most surprisingly, could have happily stayed longer. In a cave!

This kind of research has been going on since the 1930s and was even adopted by NASA to test how resilient human beings can be in different environments, even away from Earth. And through all the studies, we discovered that our bodies actually run to their own internal schedule completely separate to our external environment. This is referred to as our 'endogenous clock', and our own timing is called our 'circadian rhythm'.

The average endogenous clock runs for about 24 hours and 15 minutes. Some of us run shorter clocks and some longer, but all of us in some way need to keep recalibrating our internal clock to keep in time with the external world. A world that, in the name of convenience, runs on 9 to 5 but with 24-hour shops, gyms and restaurants. A world that stops for breakfast, lunch and dinner. The system is wide awake, the lights are always on and we have even coined new catchphrases to define what's around us: New York is the city that never sleeps.

The sun (natural light) is the most reliable signal in our environment that we set our internal clocks to. When the sun is up we are awake, if it's dark we want to sleep. Light is a huge factor in influencing our circadian rhythm. It is sunlight, more specifically blue or short wavelength light, that stimulates specific cells in the back of our eyes (called melanopsin) to send signals to our key hormone distributor, the suprachiasmatic nucleus (SCN). This sits in the brain just behind our eyes and above our pineal gland, and it's a key part of the brain's communication system. It magically synchronises the time of day with the tilt or turning of the Earth so we are drowsy at night and alert during the day, and it adjusts through the seasons.

The suprachiasmatic nucleus acts as our chief clock and is responsible for releasing hormones that signal to the body it's time to activate a specific function (it's time to wake, sleep, eat, move). It uses melatonin as its main hormone to create rhythm and keep the body in time. It interacts with many regions in the brain, including the brain stem which does most of the heavy lifting in generating sleep cycles.

In 1984, three researchers realised that actually every single cell in our body has its internal clock too. We refer to these as peripheral clocks and these are known to have a bit of a mind of their own. So now not only our system has to stay in sync with our outside world, but the Chief Conductor also needs to reign in these peripheral clocks and keep them in sync. Being out of sync creates disorganisation in our body which causes havoc on our system and robs us of energy.

The Sleep-Wake cycle is probably the most researched aspect of our circadian rhythms so our internal timing has now been mapped out in great detail offering an abundance of knowledge to use to our advantage. It is now understood that over a period of 24 hours our bodies run various levels of activity that rise and fall at peak times. During this cycle nearly every aspect of our biology shifts its duties affecting our vitals, behaviour, energy, performance and hormones, these too increasing and decreasing in a delicate see-saw balance.

Most of us have heard of the rise and fall of the Melatonin hormone. Melatonin builds up over a period of two to three hours to alert the brain it is now officially dark and is time to go to sleep. Many think of Melatonin as a natural sleeping pill, something that induces sleep, yet this hormone is just part of a communication system. Melatonin needs to build up enough in the system to signal the beginning of dark but also when it's morning and it's time to wake up. Imagine a sprinter ready to run a 100-metre race. Professor Phyllis C Zee describes melatonin as being the starting gun that tells the runner it's time to go, no what makes the athlete run.

The Cortisol hormone, our 'I'm alert' hormone, begins to rise as Melatonin wanes – waking our system up, slowly increasing our blood pressure, our body temperature and priming us to finally get out of bed.

The hormone that actually makes us feel sleepy is Adenosine and it's tightly linked to our energy production and activity levels. Adenosine doesn't kick in just before bed and send us to sleep in a jiffy, rather it builds up in our system over the course of the day, gradually creating what we refer to as sleep pressure, the desire to fall asleep.

In an ideal world, you'd be active during the day, steadily building just the right amount of sleep pressure (Adenosine) to take you to dusk when Melatonin tells you it's time to go to sleep, Cortisol magically decreases and you sleep like a baby for eight hours, waking up by your internal alarm clock feeling refreshed. Right. Except too many external factors start to play and cheekily remix this cocktail of hormones to create havoc in our system.

Heading home from a long day at work where he had to sit through countless meetings and push through deadlines, Chris is stressed, tired, and his body is ready to go to sleep. But he's hungry so he digs around the fridge rustling up something he can put together as dinner. Getting comfortable on the couch, he sets himself up for the evening, remote on one side, phone on the other, bigger screen dead ahead. It's been a full-on day; hectic doesn't even describe it. He has barely had time to scratch himself. He deserves a bit of me time, winding down, downloading. The episode he is watching slides into another, this light show continues, the evening stretches out, his brain thinking it's the middle of the day. He starts to feel peckish, finds himself in front of the fridge again – salad or gelato, is it really a question? Pass the chocolate sauce! Suddenly time has got away from him, it's midnight and he has an early start. Lying in bed, he is tossing and turning, eventually falling into a restless sleep that is broken too soon by an alarm. Of course he reasons with himself, two more snoozes pass, then something jogs his memory of that morning meeting and he is up and out the door. Energy level: low.

We know this story all too well. So let's rewrite it from the point of view of Chris's hormones – here's how the story would go.

Chris, get off your chair and go for a walk! What? Another meeting? But you're tired. You're stressed. I'm building too much sleep pressure, slow down! Pick the salad! Pick the salad! Not another episode. It's late, stop shining artificial light in your eyes or how is Melatonin ever going to tell you it's time to go to sleep? What now?

Gelato? Seriously? At this time of night? You're going to wake up and then we need to get the digestive system working when it's already asleep. Oh that will annoy Melatonin no end. Cortisol will be up there too. Okay come on, time to sleep. Try harder. Now wake up. Wake up. WAKE UP! Melatonin help me out here. Adenosine is still high. Doesn't he know Adenosine needs eight hours sleep to break down? We barely got five. What? No breakfast? Straight to another meeting? No more sitting please. I'm already tired just thinking about tonight's routine.

You're starting to form a clear picture here. It's really simple: what we decide to do (external factors) directly impacts our communication system, our hormones. And if we mess with our hormones (our signalling system) we mess with the sleep/wake cycle, our internal clock, our rhythm and ultimately our energy.

Our circadian rhythm has been researched at length and we now have a clear idea of when our bodies are at their prime to exercise, refuel, be awake, sleep, eat and even think. This is awesome news for your Athlete Within. By paying attention to your own circadian rhythm and tuning the timing dial you are able to optimise your energy level and get the most out of the day (and night).

Again, I want to give you some suggestions to help you stay in sync with your natural rhythm and give your Athlete Within the best chance to feel energised and ready to play hard.

Finding your rhythm

Your circadian rhythm is all about timing, so let's look at your 'when': when it's best to sleep, eat and move so you can maximise your dashboard:

- Begin with your sleep–wake cycle – aim to go to bed and wake up at the same time each day, even on weekends, or within a

30-minute buffer zone. This can take anywhere between a few days to a few weeks to get on track.

- Wake up, open up the blinds, grab some morning light, maybe catch a sunrise, take off your sunglasses (you still look cool). Maybe take a 20-minute walk in the early morning light (get outside). This is when blue light is at its highest, a great way to help you sync your circadian rhythm.

- Your body tends to release more insulin in the morning hours so aim to eat more at breakfast and lunch and stay lighter at dinner.

- Caffeine is a stimulant that can be found in many foods (hello chocolate). It is very sneaky as it masks your adenosine receptors, the hormones that create sleep pressure during the day. What this means is that caffeine tricks you into false (high) energy levels and then makes you crash when the effect evaporates. Keep this to a minimum, and more in the earlier part of the day, as your body takes six to eight hours to break it down.

- It is in the afternoon we reach our peak, with muscle coordination in its prime around 3 pm and muscle strength around 5 pm. These are the more ideal times to exercise. Maybe you could take a later lunch break and use that time for your training schedule. Research is telling us exercising into the night wakes us up, increasing our core body temperature, putting us more on alert and less likely to fall asleep.

- Stop eating at least three hours before your head hits the pillow, or more – the time for eating is during the day. Research is now leaning towards nighttime fasting, suggesting a window of eight to twelve hours where we don't eat and then break the fast with breakfast. This way our body has plenty of time to regenerate and increase energy. This routine has already made the mainstream, known as the Wolverine diet as one of the elements Hugh Jackman employs to develop his incredible physique.

- As darkness falls we tend to switch on the lights and lengthen our days. So to keep you in sync, you can dim blue lights and opt for softer, warmer yellow light.
- If you're wanting to use screens at night, consider blue blocker glasses – you will also look way cooler. Also look at the settings on your devices to lower the brightness and switch to warmer light.
- Consider what kind and amount of medications you are taking and whether it is more appropriate to take them at a different time of the day – a discussion to have with your GP.

Exercise

As you get familiar with your internal clock, what does your day look like? Is your circadian rhythm in sync?

Journaling is a powerful way to uncover your own unique characteristics. Write down your sleep and wake times over the next 10 days. Do they match? Are they out of sync?

Do you pay attention to the amount of light you are exposed to in the morning and at night? Are you addicted to using a screen before you go to bed?

Are the nighttime munchies part of your routine? At night, can you go eight or even ten hours without eating any food? What would it take to change these eating habits?

DIAL 5: HOW TO GET YOUR MOVEMENT RIGHT

'Nothing happens until something moves.'

Albert Einstein

Movement is definitely one of my favourite energy dials. At the end of the day, we're getting to the heart of rediscovering your Athlete Within. This book is all about getting you to reconnect to that part of you that wants to be active and embrace movement at any age. This dial is the simplest one – everyone can move at any minute of the day (and night for that matter) and it doesn't require any equipment or even much thought: we can just move. Yet this is also the hardest dial to tweak because, let's face it, we sit most of the day and then we go home to relax and sit in front of the television. We do not create much space for movement. We are often tired, sometimes unmotivated, and moving to inject energy into your body seems to be the biggest contradiction.

But to me, movement means life and it is energy. We move when we breathe. We move when we sleep. We move to stay alive. And in movement we find the key to longevity. In fact, I think this dial is so important that I cover it in much greater detail in the next step.

The equation is simple. When you move and move with purpose, your energy level goes up. And you can affect all the other dials. You sleep better, you breathe better, you eat better, you burn energy better, you perform better, you are at your best. When you move you can change your mood, your mindset, your thoughts. You can shift situations and find solutions to problems. You can break patterns and rewrite your story.

Movement is your birthright and it should not be taken for granted but used and nurtured to build your future and get you closer to your dream life. Because moving and being active is the heart of your Athlete Within.

Notes

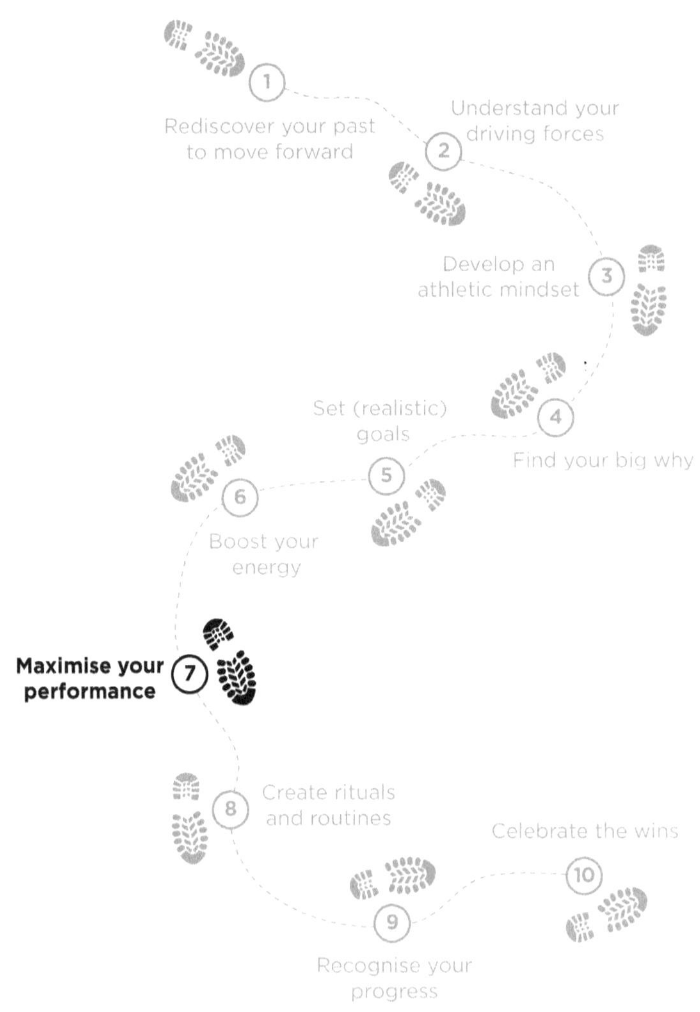

1
Rediscover your past to move forward
Understand your driving forces
2
Develop an athletic mindset
3
4
Set (realistic) goals
Find your big why
6
5
Boost your energy
Maximise your performance
7
8
Create rituals and routines
Celebrate the wins
10
9
Recognise your progress

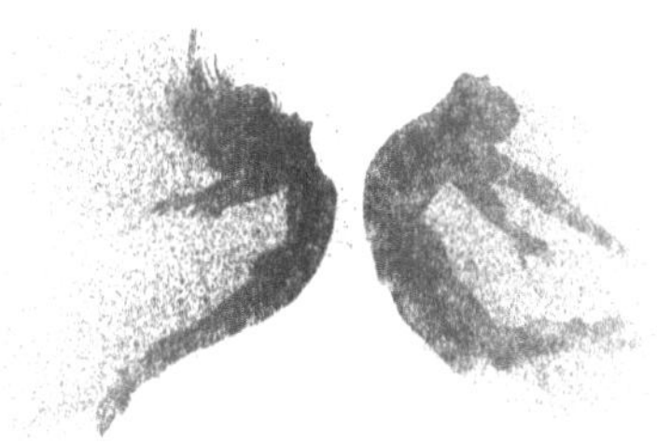

STEP 7:
MAXIMISE YOUR PERFORMANCE

MOVEMENT IS KEY TO PERFORMANCE

Inside all of us is an athlete, an idea, a dream, a talent, a flare or even desire to do something, become something. The first step is taking action. Performance begins with participation. We have all learnt the process of riding a bike, beginning with the training wheels. But training wheels slow us down and make it hard to turn, and we begin the dream of one day having more freedom. Every time we are on the bike, we are making calculations, testing them out, putting ideas into action. We return again, having processed the lessons of the last ride, refined and consolidated them in our heads, ready to put in our all, each time edging a little closer towards our target. There is no time line; it is all at our own pace.

Then one day, off come the training wheels. The first ride is never smooth, but inside you feel you have reached a new level. It's just a matter of time till you add speed, ride with no hands and pop a wheelie. This is just another step of the process, of harnessing your abilities, finding a way and performing at the next level.

If performance is ingrained in movement then movement is the language of your body. Knowing how a movement should feel and what you are trying to say is the key to good performance. If you think about language it is made up of grammar, full of rules to make sense, tied in with expression, to give it feeling. Language is further built from the spoken and the unspoken. Just like your Athlete Within there are things which seem obvious. We all come to the table with some level of understanding of what performance is, yet there is also the mystery, the unspoken that brings your athlete to life.

In this step I will walk you through understanding how we move, internalise the philosophy of slow burn, examine programming and maximising recovery, as well as developing more of who we are, a mix of awareness and perception, in the biological gym. In a world where doing less, being sedentary and seeking comfort and leisure are a short reach away, your ability to connect with deeper meaning in your own performance is crucial to the quality of life of your PM years. This is because, as Bessel van der Kolk says, 'the body keeps the score'.

FUNCTIONAL TRAINING

'You can't steal second base with your foot on first base.'

Author Frederick B. Wilcox

You're getting older, the kids have moved out, work is slowing down and you've got a little more time on your hands. Golf? Why not, it seems to be the thing, let's give it a go. You go online, buy some clubs from recommendations a golfer friend made, and – yes – you're wearing only one glove. You head out to the driving range, purchase a bucket of balls, find your own space, and you are on your way.

The first shot is pretty good, the second not too bad either, but following that it is clearly a disaster. Heading home you think, *I've got to get a coach, it's the only way I'm going to work this out before I turn 90.* Your friend gives you a name, and you make an appointment for Tuesday the following week.

The day has come. You are a little excited, but more nervous about hitting the ball in front of someone who knows their stuff. You know it doesn't make sense as you are new to this. You strike up a conversation with your coach. He cuts to the chase; let's start by seeing where you are at. You knock off a few balls, pointing out your difficulties with each shot. His silence is a bit off putting. He then moves in to help. The first thing he is doing is adjusting your posture, correcting your frame, opening your shoulders. You're bent forward, so he lifts your head, setting up a base. 'Feel where you are and own this first,' he says. This new set up is awkward and strange. Now you can't hit the ball. What does this guy really know anyway?

He begins talking to you about how form starts with your posture. 'You can't swing when you are all closed in', and something about opening up your body and being more stable, being connected to the ground. Only then you are able to breathe and relax into the shot. Feeling like a robot, you try to breathe, shake out your shoulders, resume this new position, but still he leans over to again correct your head. 'Look where you want the ball to go and then hold that thought in your mind.' You repeat to yourself this new mantra. You take the shot, and then you look up. Sailing through the air is your ball, only this time it is straight ahead, landing just to the left of the 150-metre marker, like a pro. You look at the coach, a little bewildered. All this, by just changing your body posture, using your frame, grounding yourself? The coach smiles: 'We have to start with you, not the ball.' How you approach the ball begins with how you move through space, how you hold yourself. 'You are the one swinging the club ... we all get fooled by the ball.'

Movement is orchestrated by the brain, but the brain has its own priorities that may not appear clear in the moment. Our attention may be on the wrong thing, unaware of all the activity that goes on behind the scenes to keep the show on the road. All of this is kept in check by feedback loops, updating not just where to move your hand or foot, but the knowledge of where it is in the first place. For your brain, knowing where you are in space, your orientation to the ground and anticipation of what may come are key ingredients to your performance. Your frame is the scaffolding keeping you upright, your form is your ability to control the structure not just statically but through each phase of your movement. Form and flow begin in your frame. We move our body to perform an activity. Ask a dancer – they intuitively know this already. You don't hit a ball with your wrist or hand, you move your body in to swing and hit the ball. Watch someone step up to the plate in baseball. They don't lean into the game or poke at the ball; their body is poised, ready to strike. So where do you start? Start at the beginning.

Unless you live under a rock, you have watched Roger Federer play tennis at some point. What you have witnessed is someone who embodies functional training, developing high levels of skill in the way he moves his body. A key characteristic of functional training is your ability to isolate a movement. Your ability to sense the weight of the racquet, the spring of the strings, your distance from the line and at the same time be aware of where each segment of your body is moving in high-definition detail. This ability to read your body is referred to as 'mapping'; our brains are constantly mapping what we are doing, what is happening around us and most of all constantly updating the accuracy of our map. The more accurate the detail, the faster we keep it updated, just like a computer. The faster we can read the play the faster we can respond with precision to each shot. Any glitches in our mapping lead to errors that can show up as a slip, a misfire or worse a strain or injury. We all run these maps but ours sometimes get a bit blurry or scratched, leaving us feeling clumsy and inadequate. Yet the more we give deliberate attention, hone in and keep coming back, the more we are learning, developing our library of experience and also keeping it updated.

For Federer, his skill isn't just in hitting the ball; it is his ability to relax between shots. In completely letting his system return to its state of readiness, he is enabling himself to anticipate and spring, then fully commit himself into the next shot. Practising relaxation is a key part to functional training, not just making the shot. Our muscles recruit more of their team to meet the demand, like an army. When we finish making the shot, our ability to disarm and return back to the start, our relaxed state, is called the 'relaxation moment'. If we hold tension in a part of our body, we lose energy, decreasing our capacity to anticipate, respond and move into the next play.

Each movement follows a cycle, having a set up, the activity, a follow through then the relaxation moment, where our body ideally returns to its resting state.

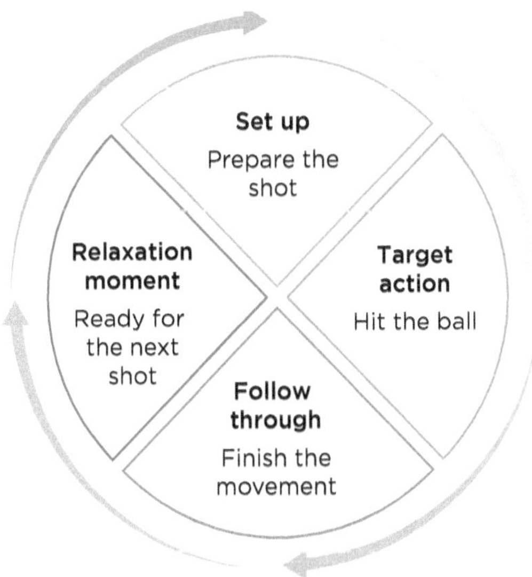

If we are not returning to a state of relaxation we are carrying tension with us from the previous shot and we are still committed from the previous play, causing two things:

· As we carry tension in our system, we limit our movement and ability to play the next shot.

· We create a habit, a 'learnt error', that with time – if not corrected – may lead to poor performance and begin to set up a pattern of repetitive injury.

Consider Federer and his training program. He was one of the longest playing competitors on the circuit, a testament to his ability to train and read his body, developing quality maps to perform ideal patterns of movement. Often in our performance we overestimate, trying too hard to achieve something as our brain is always thinking survival, playing safe, going with what is more seemingly predictable and keeping something left in the tank in case Mother Nature throws a surprise at us.

For the Athlete Within, developing awareness such as the ability to relax is often the starting point. With my clients we talk about what is effective functional training, highlighting three pillars:

· capacity and what your resources are
· your competence in what you are doing
· endurance and sustainability.

We begin with the concept of optimising movement, not building muscles, by prioritising awareness before strength or endurance.

Effective performance training begins with where you are now, determining your baseline within your parameters. With my clients this is a personalised program that includes starting points, fundamental pillars to work on, milestones and touchpoints plus defining expectations. It begins with an analysis of the individual characteristics of where you find yourself and your habitat.

Exercise

Where are you starting from? What does your routine look like? What does your day-to-day activities consist of? What are your challenges (short and long term)? What are your limitations or obstacles? Do you feel confident moving forward? Is there a plan or strategy?

Now we move on to training your Athlete Within, in three areas where we are going to get the best runs on the board: capacity, competence and endurance.

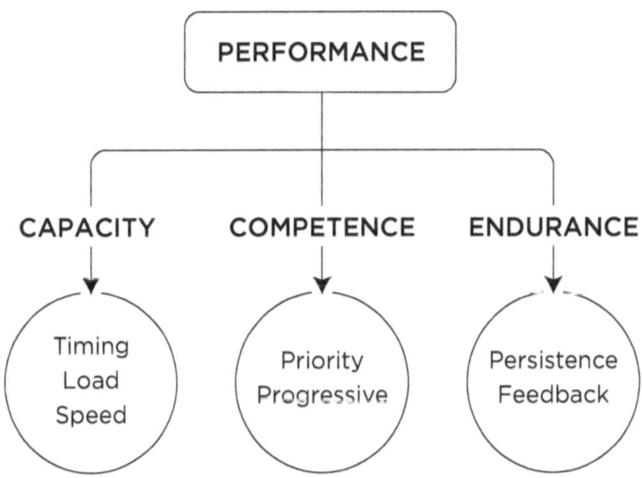

Capacity is a key focus, especially in the earlier stages looking at how resourceful you are. It is always a tough one to master – we often overestimate or underestimate our ability and what's in the tank. It is important to assess where you are right now so you know what activity you can start doing, and most importantly if you can sustain it.

To work on your capacity you can look at three key parts:

- *Timing:* Timing is your ability to control and coordinate within a situation. It is a key step to begin with, often under the banner of technique. Timing is about breaking down the way you move, working on an element of your movement pattern in isolation and then integrating it into a sequence (remember the golf swing? First the person then the ball).

- *Load:* Load is the intensity with which we train. Here we look more at frequency and repetition; how much can your body withstand when you train? Too little and you don't progress, too much and the system is overloaded and buckles.

- *Speed:* The speed of your training represents your own pace. In slowing things down you increase your attention, pick up more nuances and work the detail. Speed is also linked to how well you are progressing. Slow and steady? Too fast and crashing it? As we dive deeper into performance, you'll see how pace becomes more of an approach to each facet of the Athlete Within and what we apply our attention to (slow burn).

Competence is how well you can do something and your ability to learn, improve and progress. It's an integral part of functional training as it focuses on building proficiency and confidence, giving you momentum to carry on. When you work on your competence, think of how you prioritise and if you are progressing:

- *Priority:* This is about directing your attention exactly where it needs to go: what is your order and sequence in your training? What do you start your training with? And what ritual do you finish with? For your Athlete Within this is about not getting lost in the woods, but keeping your attention free and focused either on the 'one thing' or your top three priorities.

- *Progressiveness:* Functional training must always be progressive, particularly from an emotional point of view, which is tied up in your reward system and your will to follow through.

The last area for you to consider is **Endurance**. Endurance is having enough to go all the way. It's about building habits during your training that will help you achieve your goals, improve and continue to move forward. Endurance requires you to be persistent and in tune with your body, knowing how to adjust, tweak and overcome:

- *Persistence:* Persistence is repetition built over time. It reinforces habits towards excellence, improving the profile and repertoire of your training one step at a time.

- *Feedback:* Reading your body and yourself is a key to knowing where you are at and when to flex. You can give yourself feedback daily or weekly or even during a performance, being a measure of your energetic flow.

The beauty of rediscovering your Athlete Within is that you only need to focus on one of these elements and build it in time, making it yours, before you go to the next.

Here's a little list of exercises you can work with towards capacity, competence and endurance to help you improve your performance:

- **Floor work:** Working from the floor is a great way to begin isolation training. It enables you to remove complexity and put more deliberate attention to aspects of your technique. Keep it simple. Be clear on what part of your movement you are isolating and feel when you are doing it correctly. If you are going it alone, a great place to start is with Professor Stuart McGill's 'Big 3' exercises. They're very similar to the ones I use with my clients and you can easily find them online.

- **Awareness training:** I love gentle rhythmic stretching that is slow (rather than static), taking the body through its range of motion. This can include tai chi, chi gong, yoga or similar modalities. They are coordinated disciplines that focus on slow, flowing movement and creating awareness. In this step I often add a small home trampoline to add rhythmic bouncing to a program.

- **Visual training:** Optic flow is a key part of our Athlete Within performance, integrating vision with movement. We start with training hand–eye coordination. It can be as simple as walking while bouncing and catching a handball.

- **Dynamic training:** Advancing from floor work, we are now building complexity into your movement. More than increasing the difficulty or intensity of an exercise, here we want to add layers of movement to the way you exercise. This shifts you from using linear, predictable patterns to movements that are more complex, such as twisting and going side to side. It's like adding dimensions to your movement patterns so your Athlete Within can learn to be more dynamic, more responsive, more whole. It could be incorporating a tri-planar style exercise, developed by Gary Grey, or simply going for a walk up a hill that involves a new terrain and changing directions.

Exercise

Dig into the vast menu of possibilities we've just explored and pick one. Work on one aspect of your performance. Maybe keep a record so you can review, tick off items on the list and track your progress.

THE PRINCIPLE OF SLOW BURN

Slow Burn is a book that introduces ideas Stu Mittleman embraced as part of his ultra-running success. For me personally, slow burn grew as a concept in my clinic. It was a way to program people and work to timeframes, but as my knowledge grew in the world of chronic pain, slow burn became more of a philosophy – there is always an answer if we keep working.

The concept of slow burn affected the way I thought about practising as well as how I would onboard clients coming into my clinic. It was a theme that took many directions. Working at a spinal level people always wanted the quick fix. I would tell them there are two doors here: the first one is about getting rid of pain, it is a quick option and tends to be a revolving door where we will keep meeting again and again, or there is a second door where you get involved, work with me and realise it has taken years for you to reach this point where your spine has buckled and it is going to take time to recondition yourself.

All too often we overestimate, then overload and overwhelm ourselves. Feeling defeated, we stop, barely, only to return to the desire we began with in the first place. Rather than someone putting us through our paces, showing us the bigger picture and telling us it's all about sticking with it and giving it the time it needs, we jump at the quick fix and then become despondent when it does not work. Training follows the same principle.

Every new learning needs to go through its seasons before it becomes part of us. We have to experience not just the honeymoon and excitement of spring and then move into the summer months. We also need to experience difficulty, challenge and conflict as we move into the autumn and winter months, where the end isn't always clear. With time and holding onto a belief, we survive, we live through the seasons, we mature and develop the growth rings that come with experience and understanding.

Slow burn is a philosophy about not only awareness of who you are as your Athlete Within but finding your own pace, staying in your own lane, and learning to work with your own body conditions. The meaning of slow burn is in the word: burn slowly. To maximise your performance you need to give yourself time to truly go through every step, without rushing. You build endurance one brick at a time. Slowly. With deliberate intention. Learning the ropes. Making it yours. Just as you approach the 10 steps in this book. Going through the exercises. Making the last one count so you can build on the next.

Slow burn isn't so much a 'doing' step but more a 'step back and think' step. It is realising your Athlete Within isn't a destination but has destinations along the road. That meeting these is not just the achievement, but also the enjoyment, and the spirit it brings makes us who we are. This is considering the bigger picture and how we go about the thinking of our Athlete Within. Often we put so many pressures and expectations on ourselves.

Your Athlete Within is about making decisions with you as the priority. Time is on your side. Slow burn is about setting your own pace, reading your own body and self, checking in and making it last. There are many lessons that can be learnt from the ultra-athlete within.

THE RECOVERY FACTOR

Remember the story from the opening of the book about Professor Stuart McGill, being stronger and training more effectively at the age of 78 than in his 50s? Much of this he puts down to recovery, the ability to not only change gears but to use each of our gears effectively. Recovery is a key to your performance. We can't be ON all the time running at top speed. We aren't machines, but at the same time recovery is not a day off, it's like the yin needs the yang. Recovery emphasises organising your rituals and sticking to them.

In my 20s training with a group of triathletes, they would have spin days on the bike, often following a high-intensity session the day before. Heading out, it was more a social ride in my mind, pedalling at a very slow and casual pace, not a lot of kilometres, a leisurely day out, spinning the wheels. But really it was a meeting on the road, revisiting the previous day's highlights or learnings, reinforcing the movement, just doing it in a way that didn't stress their bodies. To my young mind it was a pure waste of time; I could be putting in another big session, building some serious kilometres and improving my speed, or working a hill and making the most of the day.

Add on 25 years of clinical experience, my attitude has changed 180 degrees and solidified through my conversations with Professor McGill. Recovery can be used to increase the feeling, the knowledge and understanding of the conditions.

Recovery calls for deliberate attention, working in a lower gear with a different intensity and a different end goal in mind. This is also applied to your performance programming: putting deliberate attention to the activity you do day in day out. When you run the same five kilometres you improve at first but quickly reach a plateau, your body becomes used to it, it knows what to expect and it's not challenged enough. This leads to loss of condition and strength. Mix it up: different terrain, different speed, different length…get creative, trick your body, sharpen the sword.

Recovery is still going through the motions but without the load. Your body has a chance to repair and catch up, while still continuing the learning and staying in the game. Often when we learn a new movement, in the beginning it is quite fragile. It's not the breathing or the physical movement that is the limiting factor – it is our brain getting its head around it, working it out so that we can repeat it and improve. Your recovery is moving through each level of the gears of your Athlete Within.

Recovery has three aspects:

- grooving
- priming
- sleeping.

Training your groove is skill development, working the right movement habits. Priming the system is knowing the feeling of your sweet spot and your ability to produce it. Getting the right sleep matters because at night your brain is working its different gears and reinforces movement patterns learnt during the day.

Grooving (repetition)

When we are grooving we are repeating and reinforcing a characteristic pattern of movement that directly relates to our Athlete Within, learning the moves until they become second nature. Learning is effectively clocking up the hours in a deliberate way. You are going through the motions, decreasing your tissue load, by travelling at a lower speed but feeling the movement in your body. In running or swimming you are practising a particular stride or stroke and honing understanding of the particular characteristics that are applicable and the feeling of the movement across the terrain or through the water until you reach the point where you just own it. In recovery grooving, you are changing to a lower gear but continuing the characteristic movement.

When I think about tissue stress, the word that pops into my mind is 'tolerance'.

Tolerance is the story of loading and demand, how much the tissues in your body can handle before micro-tearing takes effect, the tug-of-war of stress versus strain. Generally we think about this as a muscle thing. We are all familiar with waking up the following day with stiffness and tired muscles, or worse two days later when we can't walk up the stairs (delayed muscle onset). Tolerance relates also to your ligament and fascial systems, made up of connective tissue, primarily collagen. After sitting at a desk all day, inactivity creeps in and these connective tissue layers are in more of a state of fatigue. Hitting the yoga studio after work – taking your body through a number of movements – accelerates reaching your tolerance point, opening the door to the onset of injury. This is where grooving recovery is key, building up your tolerance not only to that kind of characteristic movement but also the time of day you choose – remember that circadian thing? Even for our bones there is a tolerance point, reached often with endurance or repetition of a particular movement such as a stress fracture.

Walking the line of injury, a discussion on tolerance is more than just how you feel today, but journaling the highs and lows to distinguish and tease out the elements more crucial to monitor. Having had a lot of experience with spinal disc injuries, often the best thing to do in these cases is to keep moving rather than rest, using a strategy of micro-breaks, correct movement management (such as getting in and out of a chair) and amount of recommended activity. No pain doesn't equate to no problem, it just takes you through one door into the next, still requiring a strategy to assess degree, type of activity and progress.

Groove training is an art that needs to be worked to find your individuality, beginning with decreased load and increased diversity. Pulling back on the accelerator and lowering the speed is easy to grasp, yet the nuances are more about moving with less effort and finding a different rhythm. I start people by decreasing one aspect to 30% effort and discussing what this means, how they can measure and then, importantly, reading their body, knowing what to look for to gauge how their body is running. When unsure, drop it. Running may drop to speed walking, speed walking may drop to a slow walk when you listen to the body. Remember the focus here is taking out the physical load and moving the body along the lines of your Athlete Within characteristics.

Diversifying is another option. Working the body in a different way means you are feeding the movement to the body in a different manner, shifting the movement to a different part of the body. The key to grooving diversity is being curious enough to find a movement that is different from the primary movement pattern yet still relatable to the profile of your Athlete Within. In swimming, rather than freestyle, your recovery might be using your kickboard. You're still in the pool with the feeling of moving through water but you're diverting the concentration of effort to a different part of your body

Priming (being deliberate)

Priming emphasises the mental learning preparation for your athlete in your recovery gear, paying more attention to the feeling of performance. Priming is about combining information from the environment, internal and external, with being in the right place at the right time, your sweet spot, with the rhythm of movement. Moving into your recovery gear, priming is slowing down your performance, replaying it, working the nitty-gritty details. Essentially priming is about your readiness.

A short but key point to remember is that even your brain needs recovery. Our noisy world can at times be too much. I like to find solitude, silence and stillness walking along the beach to the sounds of crashing waves. Clients in my clinic have often expressed the joy of a game of golf to help them relax but also still move while in recovery mode. There are times when we want to distance ourselves and step back. We can feel our heart just isn't in it; something as simple as procrastination may be a signal for you to change mental gears.

Priming could be taking a shot in slow motion, walking rather than running the terrain, familiarising yourself with difficult or transition points, with your accountability buddy or coach. This could be modelling, strategising in motion or visualisation. The great ice hockey player Wayne Gretzky 'wasn't big enough, strong enough or even fast enough' – his magic came from watching games on TV and seeing the underlying patterns and flow of the game, teaching himself to skate to where the puck was going. As we are creatures of habit, priming gives clear instructions to help build and tune your feeling of being at your fullest in the sweet spot, quickly finding your state of readiness.

Priming recovery is shifting your groove attention more to technique and fundamentals. Michael Jordan would rehearse layups for hours after everyone else had gone home. Even a kid starting basketball begins here; it is the ABCs of basketball, but only the greats realise that time invested in this low gear can pay off at intense times of a game.

One of my passions is trail running, but occasionally I will go to an indoor centre and invest time in climbing. It is a movement that works my body in a different way, allowing recovery. And it hones my vision of where I am going, as well as improving my body awareness to help with finding my feet on a slope.

Sleeping (cleaning and learning)

Hearing about sleep is a bit deflating. It's like being told you need to eat more veggies. But sleeping means recovery, it means cleaning and learning. Our brain has already worked out how to make the most of the dark, using the time to drain, repair, process, download, scrutinise and then consolidate learnings into your library of performance experience. Sleep is about learning and assimilating your athlete into your body. It's about getting the right amounts of the different stages of sleep (now that you are an expert on the architecture of sleep from Step 6): deep SWS (clean, repair, grow) and REM (scrutinise, consolidate, emotional assimilation).

To make a tough decision or better understand something, sleep on it. All of this is a part of modelling, but in a bigger sense it deepens the way we prime and the way we feel the movement in our body, and will increase the speed of attaining our sweet spot.

Sleep recovery is putting attention on the strategy and understanding of your Athlete Within. The essence of sleep is reinforcing concepts and ideas into your mind to gain a better overall picture of you as your athlete and the environment in which you participate.

*

Recovery not only complements, it invigorates and excites the development of your Athlete Within. Taking hold of recovery can not only help build capacity, it can help deepen the groove of learning fundamental movement and thinking. Recovery is flipping the notion of just resting – rather we are opening windows of possibility and injecting creativity by using it to learn and train in different gears and maximise our up time and down time in training.

Exercise

1. Can you find a way to decrease your load and recover? What can you do to consolidate your skills and movement at a slower pace? Maybe walk instead of run, or recover from your tennis training with a game of table tennis, enjoying the speed and hand–eye coordination it offers.

   Changing gears may be investing time in breathing exercises and some stability floor work.

2. Why not challenge yourself and sign up for ballet classes for one term, just to feel your body move in a different way and look for insights that relate to your own athlete?

3. Spend some time before you go to sleep imagining yourself performing a particular move or technique as your Athlete Within. Feel how you want to move, fine tuning elements

or a new technique, ironing out the creases and cutting the groove deeper.

GET INTO THE BIOLOGICAL GYM

Hiking through Tasmania is an experience – a delicate ecosystem surrounded by ragged mountains that leaves you breathless, especially when the sun moves through the sky to mark the end of another day, the light giving a display difficult for a photo to truly capture. The horizon stretches forever over the ocean, the lightning in the distance indicating a storm brewing. A scampering in the grass off to the side pulls you back to where you stand, leaving you wondering what else is in your vicinity. Even the different fungi, their range of colours, seem to cause a sense of wonder. Time spent outdoors, just you and nature, seems to sharpen our senses, quietens us, causing us to turn more inwards as we take all this in.

Even half an hour from Sydney and you can be in the bush, easily finding your own track to get lost in. An uneven fire trail or walking track quickly becomes your rugged playground. Away from the noise of the roads and traffic, out of sight of square buildings, you find yourself having a relationship with nature. Getting to know the feel of the terrain, the twists and turns, the awkward tilt of the trail, the branches on the path, the boulders you step over as you navigate your way through each of these obstacles. Then there is being outdoors in the sun, soaking up its warmth, the quiet allowing you to get lost in your own thoughts. All of this unwinding you of the pressures you find yourself in. It is just you, the terrain and the conditions, sharing nature with the birds, and a random echidna or wallaby.

There is something about being outside in Mother Nature that seems to draw us away from the worries and difficulties of this modern life. Whether it is the openness, the variety of colours, the intense smells, the sound of birds or the bright sun on our faces as we walk through the bush, it just seems to transport us to a different place inside ourselves, shifting the very essence of our being. Time in the outdoors energises us and reconnects us, leaving us feeling rejuvenated and ready to head back and face our own worlds.

Of course for us homo sapiens, the outdoors or wilderness is where we spent our ancestral childhood. We had a more physical way of life, growing up in the elements of nature, under the stars, tinkering away with our various ideas, shaping our destiny. Standing the test of time, ice ages, famine, disease – yet through it all we survived, adapted and thrived, exploring lands, navigating our way across oceans to other continents, conquering just about every ecosystem, every nook on planet Earth.

Our modern way of life is of concrete, hard, straight, narrow paths with ninety-degree corners. Our vision is hampered by rising blocks of buildings, all a far cry from the wilderness we once knew. The comforts and luxuries seem to dull our senses. Nature is so rich in its complexities, from the uneven ground dotted with its irregular rocks and tree roots to paths that trail off and become lost among trees. To hike means staying alert, lifting your knees so as not to trip on the edge of a loose rock or slippery surface, all the while keeping your attention not at your feet but on where you are heading.

The biological gym can play a part in developing your Athlete Within, a key ally in building awareness before strength and endurance. It is where developing plasticity and adaptability come in. It is not a recipe or a section out of a textbook, it is a feeling. Working with the terrain is working with this feeling, knowing it, understanding it, growing it and being able to access it easily. Your awareness is built on blending your inner intelligence with experience. The terrain is your teacher, telling you to lift your knees, watch your step, be careful not to fall, move your body, keep your timing and keep your head up so you can see where you are going. Nature is the ultimate gym to help develop, shape and sharpen your performance.

With adding the biological gym into people's programs, their Athlete Within blossomed. They increased awareness that improved their ability to isolate movement segments. They improved their timing which reduced injury. They improved their stabilisation and their confidence in their own performance. The unpredictability and complexity of the terrain became another construct for learning movement and performance. The increased stimulation led to increased activation in their body and alertness in their minds, bringing about better ability in their response, improving their overall performance.

Exercise

Create your own experience on new terrain. Organise a hike, make it an adventure. Consider something scenic, such as walking to a lookout where you can gaze into the distance and allow yourself the time to soak it all up.

Explore your local area. Search for your own terrain and begin a new journey in nature. Schedule a run or a hike. Allow yourself at least two hours, prepare well from your feet to hydration, and employ the concepts of slow burn.

The first step in learning is delicate. Your body is paying attention to a lot of new things; allow your body to develop anticipation.

One last thing: performance needs a solid structure and planning, so you can make time to work on it with purpose and in line with your goals. We are creatures of habit but making habits that stick sometimes is the hardest thing. It's time to look at your rituals and routines.

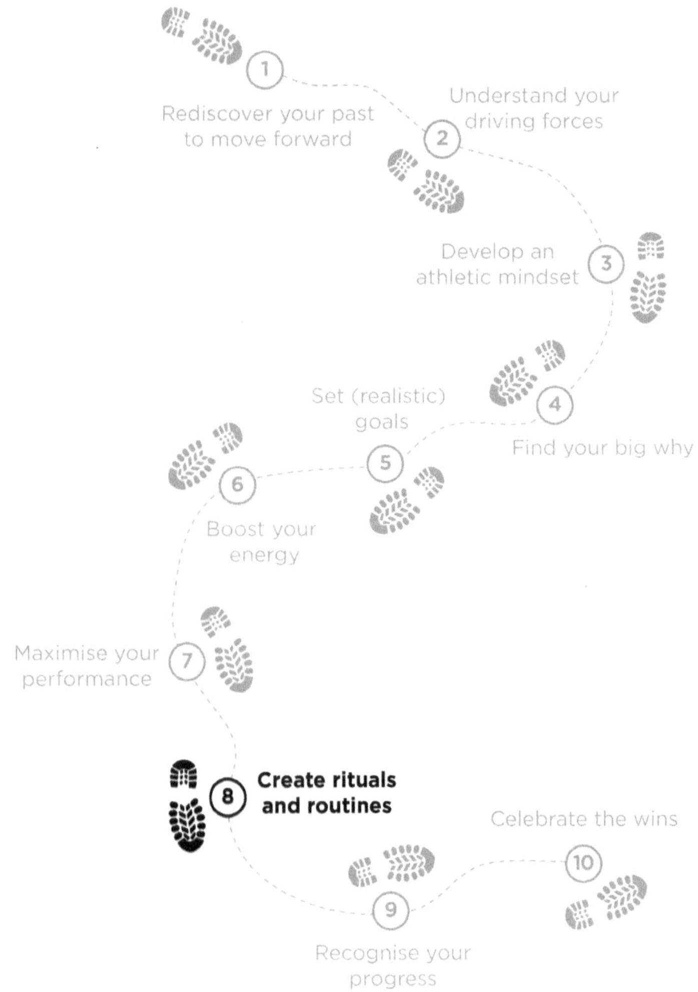

1
Rediscover your past to move forward
Understand your driving forces
2
Develop an athletic mindset
3
4
Find your big why
Set (realistic) goals
5
6
Boost your energy
Maximise your performance
7
8
Create rituals and routines
Celebrate the wins
10
9
Recognise your progress

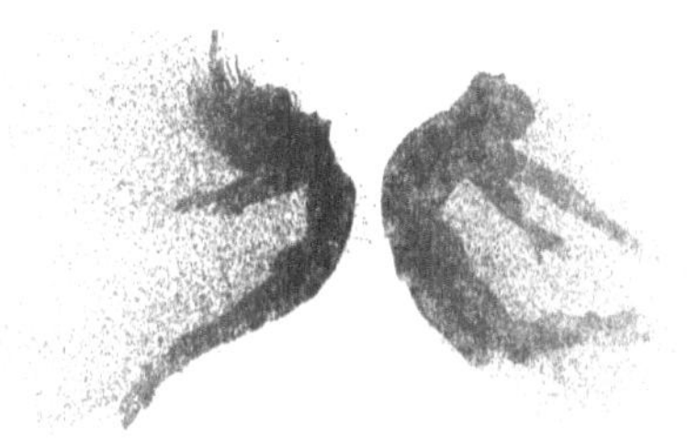

STEP 8: CREATE RITUALS AND ROUTINES

Imogen had grown up with a little bit of dance, a little bit of gymnastics and school sports, so she knew how to throw and kick a ball, but she preferred a book any day of the week. The man she married grew up loving sport, in particular soccer – one of those guys who seemed to quickly pick up anything he played. Their careers took off, and they settled into a life of routine that over the years became less and less active. The weeks seemed to race past.

Then a friend had a shock: a heart attack one Sunday night, leaving them not only upset but questioning their own level of health and their lifestyle. Of course the answer: let's join the gym. A great, ambitious project, without any further thought. And over the years there was a lot of start–stop, try another gym, attend a particular class, but the story never lasted more than two or three months.

This story now had a four-year history of well-intended repeated starting points. When I had a conversation with Imogen, she really had a lot of frustration and emotion around getting started. We worked on her why, with more detail around her goal and her feeling around the gym. Rather than it being a chore, all grind and no fun, we connected the experience more to her why, engaging her more at an emotional level. Surprisingly to her husband, she then chose boxing. She also decided to spend just seven minutes each morning punching away as part of her daily ritual to bring about more movement in her day. This in particular she enjoyed. It was short, she could do it in her pyjamas in the lounge room, she could put music on and she felt playful. Over the weeks, she was telling me how she would wake up rather than arguing with the snooze alarm, looking forward to her morning ritual. She could see her technique improve, she was sharing with members of her class and soon their chats flowed into a few weekend coffee catchups. They shared their own stories.

She had found her people, her tribe, and created her own rituals and routines that meant she was enjoying her exercise instead of see-ing it as a boring chore, and this made it much easier for her to stick to. The pattern of start–stop was over, and Imogen was on her way to her goals.

SHAPE THE WAY YOU LIVE YOUR EVERYDAY

It's our rituals and routines that make us who we are. As humans we love predictability, we fall in love with our 'ways'. But then we also love the mystery, the surprise that comes with the unpredictable.

The discipline of who you become starts with the way you live your everyday, embedded in the rituals you find yourself following. Rediscovering your Athlete Within is a process of building discipline, developing good habits and integrating these layers into your way of life and who you are becoming. To create change is to start with changing your rituals.

The overarching aim in rediscovering your Athlete Within is to transform who you are becoming. The biggest thing that will influence who you become is your habits. Changing rituals and routines begins with everyday small-scale changes, called the 'one percenters', that you apply with deliberate *attention*.

Why do we become lost in the clouds, rather than focusing on what's in front of us? Mastery begins in simplicity. Engagement is how you relate to something, how the small things fit in the bigger picture. Admiral McRaven, a retiring Navy Seal, gave an incredible commencement address in 2014 where he explained how discipline wasn't just a way of life, for a Navy Seal it was about survival. He begins with the simplicity of just making your bed every morning, a habit that was passed down to him from his peers. It wasn't about making the bed, but more about the discipline he built at the beginning of every day, the 1% that set the tone for the way he lived his life as a Navy Seal.

Discipline requires application with deliberate attention or else your Athlete Within will sink. To create lasting habits we must get excited by setting our path, placing goals along the way towards our overarching vision of our Athlete Within. We wear so many hats in life, it's easy to lose our priorities. As opportunities appear they become weighed down by less significant to-do's, so sticking to your one percenters needs a strategy. What's going to keep you in the game?

A key aspect of transforming is giving your Athlete Within time. Often this comes in the form of patience. Actor Jim Carrey once said, 'It took me sixteen years to become an overnight success'. Discipline needs time to mature and for us to reap the benefits. Applying discipline is constantly influencing ourselves over time, even when the results may not be instant or obvious. It is your ability to lead yourself from within and not give up. Rediscovering your athlete is a process of defining your version of yourself, connecting to your why root, harnessing your mindset, and setting your goals and the action steps required. Then capturing all of this and turning it into a plan, a framework of discipline, repeatedly practising your changes in a deliberate manner. It is here we embrace time as part of our expectations in a way that allows us to set ourselves up to win.

There are three phases to working on your plan to create new routines and rituals in your life:

- You begin in the more strategic, mechanical phase of working out the steps, the direction and places you will visit along the way in the form of goals.

- Then you take a step back and tinker, in particular considering what could mess this up (a point we cover more below).

- Lastly you sprinkle in time, that wonderful ingredient we often forget about till it's too late. How will you fit this in to your already busy life?

Your plan can include:

- Goals: do your goals feel real to you? Is your timeframe realistic or are you biting off more than you can chew?

- Strategies: how are you going to implement your plan? (What is it you are prioritising, making your one thing? What is the sequence of steps your need to follow?)

- Action steps: are you clear on what you are asking yourself to do? And how will you go about it?

- Timeframe: are your action steps progressive and following a sequence towards a milestone? Are you thinking long term?

- Check ins: have you scheduled ahead your 'stop-and-stare appointments' with your Athlete Within?

- Documenting: what have you got to show for yourself? Can you show your plan to someone else?

- Journalling: tell your story. Give it feeling. Describe the angst, the conflict, talk about wins, the rewards and especially how you felt.

- You can also record metrics, reflections and insights.

Key to your plan is having the belief you can do it, it is more than possible, and you feel that you own it. This begins with sharing your story with the people around you. When you tell people you love to hike, you will begin sharing hiking stories.

Your plan brings structure from which you can build and grow. It is your discipline, your rules and behaviour that will keep it relevant. Start with recognising and running with your strengths. What are you already good at? What do you enjoy? Then build from your base.

Starting this process, people tend to fall into two groups:

- those struggling to really get started and actually get the plane off the ground (like Lisa and her karate)

- those who love the dance of taking off, but over time become distracted by the chaos and conditions of life and try to shift their direction of navigation while still in the air, only to run out of fuel and quietly crash in the hinterland (like Julian and his marathon).

With this in mind, some people tend to require more time working on their structure and defining their routines (Julian), whereas for others (Lisa) beginning with their behaviours is more key, initially spending more time on their rituals. Is there one element you feel causes you the greatest conflict? Starting or carrying on?

Crafting your Athlete Within begins with discipline, setting routines and meaningful exercise. Repeat your new routine enough times till it becomes a ritual, then with maturity your brain will onboard it as a habit. As long as you keep recalibrating, it will move into autopilot and become an unbreakable habit. The discipline comes in the application, stepping boldly into our new trajectory.

Once you can see what is possible to change, you can then move towards application and implementation. By building from the ground up, you are adding in daily changes which feel easy, making it possible to repeat and enjoy the feeling of how simple the art of discipline can be.

Rituals and routines are where the rubber meets the road. We take an idea, give it a why root and an identity, design a goal path and then we hit the doing stage. The doing stage is about finding your discipline.

HOW TO SET YOURSELF UP TO WIN

This is the point you sit down and work through your plan. Preparation is setting yourself up to win, lining up all the dots and considering the possibilities to flex and anticipate. This is preparing for implementation.

Imogen initially began her gym routine following some New Year's Eve resolutions, setting goals with great intentions, but her starting and stopping was due to poor implementation of her Athlete Within process. Imogen didn't have great habits. She saw everyone else heading to the gym – they were getting into shape, so she followed the pack. But to her, the gym was a chore. She didn't connect with following the plan.

Imogen left out vital ingredients in rediscovering her Athlete Within: without a why root or a definition of her Athlete Within to connect her to her athletic pursuit she quickly became bored, looking for valid reasons why she couldn't make it to the gym that day. After spending a little time with Imogen, she began laughing about the fact she would prefer to go rollerblading than pack her bag for the gym, but she hadn't rollerbladed since she was a teenager. By going back and rediscovering her Athlete Within her story started to unfold. We did some more prep and moved into a plan. Imogen started with purchasing some rollerblades – hot pink with sequins – then skating once a week on the weekend for a minimum of two hours. Her husband was on board as her buddy, preferring his scooter for transport, and they would pick a different location each weekend to explore, take a picnic and it became her thing. Whether it was being a big kid skating again or just the hot new blades she was wearing, it quickly took off. At her three-week check-in, Imogen described how breathless she was and out of shape. So she started walking more. Her work was close to a large park. Starting with thirty minutes walking in the park easily fit in with her work, and she began walking a minimum of twice per week.

I saw Imogen three months later. She had continued her skating; now in summer, she did an afternoon skate here and there. As her activity increased, so did her energy, so did her enthusiasm, and now she had returned to the gym with a work friend. Her discipline of rollerblading once a week rubbed off on her husband, who began his own journey rediscovering his own Athlete Within. He began running beside her while she bladed. Oh, and she still does her morning boxing, in her pyjamas, in her loungeroom, to pumping music. Good habits die hard.

IMPLEMENT

Implementing is about creating your habits, the standards we live by, and focuses on:

- Small and often: the art of the one percenters.
- Make it incremental: start with what you know, work with progress and build up.
- Intensity: keep working on your base threshold or you will plateau.

What can get in the way is conflict, both internal and external, the chaos of life or what I love to call the three amigos: overwhelm, overload and overestimation. Life tends to speed up, we fall back and think on the level of to-do's, a list that never ends, and soon we are swallowed up by life and come crashing down in overwhelm. Or we are poor decision makers, and we don't turn our 'shoulds' into 'musts' until we have too many things on our plate. We try to control everything and we become overloaded. Or we don't take the time to correctly plan, and we go all out and decide to run a marathon in two months. Yet we don't update and recalibrate the path of our Athlete Within when we realise we have over-reached. We speed up, only to come crashing down again as we have overestimated. Rather than living the life we want and the joy of our Athlete Within, we get stuck and live in our heads.

There is also your outer shell to explore; in rediscovering your Athlete Within you tap into the village mentality. Often we try to do things alone rather than dipping into the wealth of resources around us. All too frequently we don't realise what's available to us until we begin to ask.

The teacher appears when the student is ready and can step out of the heat of the moment, our emotional bonds, and see the bigger picture of our Athlete Within. There are times when we have a burning question and we just need confirmation in the form of wisdom that we are moving in the right direction.

Never underestimate the power of sharing. As we tell the village we also shift our identity and set a promise in action.

In developing discipline in your rituals and routines, you can also pay attention to proximity as an outside influencer. Decorate your space, and use photos, art or music. Set signposts, whether that be a calendar, a chart with metrics or just fun reminders to inspire you along the way – whatever takes you closer towards the feeling of being your Athlete Within.

Exercise

What is it going to take for you to follow through? What rituals and routines can you set in place to beat boredom and overwhelm?

What standards do you adhere to in forming your habits?

Who are three people you can tap into to help develop the discipline required to become your Athlete Within? Schedule a meeting with them right now. What three things in particular could you ask their wisdom about?

Have you got your dream team lined up and ready to cheer you on?

As you think about your inner you and the habits you are about to embrace, are you ready to implement?

The habits of the Athlete Within are stepping stones that provide structure and bring about momentum and growth. As you make them yours, and you feel the surge of momentum, you can be confident in the knowledge that progress is happening. Now you just need to stop and recognise it.

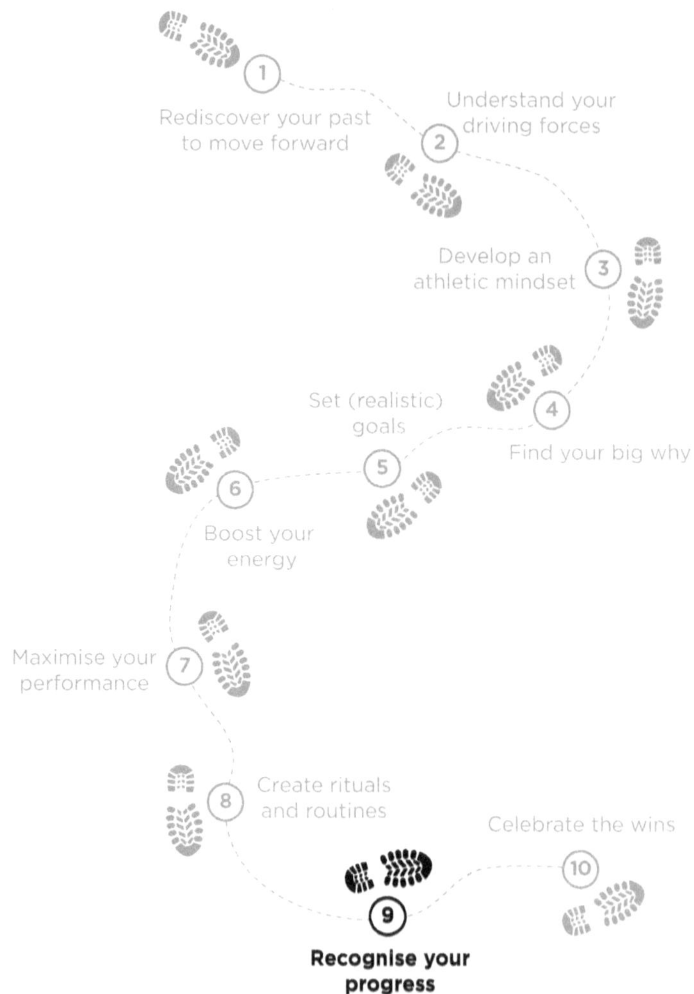

1
Rediscover your past to move forward
2
Understand your driving forces
3
Develop an athletic mindset
4
Find your big why
5
Set (realistic) goals
6
Boost your energy
7
Maximise your performance
8
Create rituals and routines
9
Recognise your progress
10
Celebrate the wins

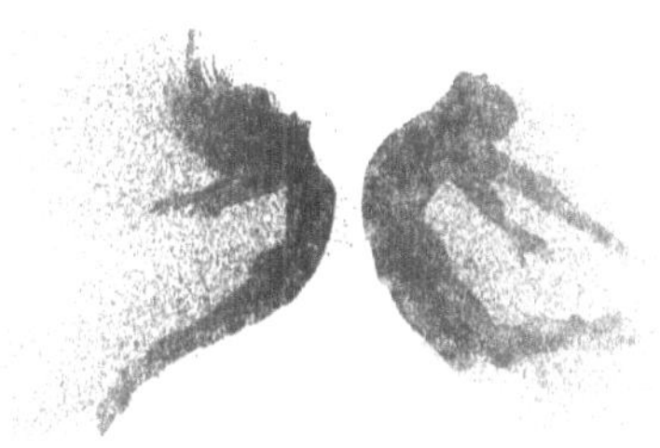

STEP 9:
RECOGNISE YOUR PROGRESS

'No one on the planet has the same experiences, trials, tribulations, realisations, battles, victories or moments as you. Use what makes you unique.'

Bestselling author Andrew Griffiths

RECOGNISING AND MASTERY

I see mastering as a delicate situation of stepping out of your story and coming at it from another angle. Your ultimate mentor is the one you find within. Life in many ways is uncovering and unwrapping who you are, becoming more you. It takes time, it takes space, it is a process, your own story. It is like stepping away from yourself, moving to the side, taking a seat and contemplating. Mastering is understanding we move towards what we are compelled to, and along the way it is important to check in and take the time to contemplate. As life unfolds, we learn more. As much as we like to figure things out on the go, there is mastery that comes about when one stops to recognise where we are in the process. There is mastery in stopping to celebrate the rewards along the way. It is said this life is a short one; but is it a life well lived?

An important aspect of your plan for developing your Athlete Within is making the time for reflection, onboarding the lessons gained but also the deeper insights that come with the combination of experience and reflection. Recognising is about running through your game plan, tweaking where needed, becoming more familiar with the big picture, questioning it, pulling and twisting it around, making it more you. All too often in life we run down a particular rabbit hole; it looks like a shortcut, you give an eager spurt, yet you run out of mojo, lose the oomph and end up facing the wrong direction. Mastery is in the adjustments you make along the journey to finetune and recalibrate, where lessons are first recognised and given due meaning and priority. Recognising is essentially making the time and space to check in on your true north.

Recognising is going through moments of evaluating, exploring, designing, crafting and remodelling our Athlete Within. Essentially we are moving through checkpoints to consider and gain insight on the road so far, as well as anticipating the adventures that may lie ahead. As we work through these checkpoints, we turn from an internal perspective to an external perspective.

We start our journey from the inside, our own perspective. We explore the interaction between chaos and order from specific points of view. The path we travel in life is rarely a straight one, often full of unforeseen potholes and difficult roads to navigate. We then move to a second checkpoint, this time utilising our external perspective, seeking wisdom from the resources we have around us, in particular our mentors or coach and accountability buddy.

Remember, you experience life in your mind first, predicting how this moment will play out, creating an expectation. When life plays our hand and our prediction is correct, we create experiences that become more automatic and habitual. When our prediction meets a mismatch we have to either recalibrate or divert. How we assess this determines how we interpret the moment and react. If we have a miss, do we become frustrated and anxious, or do we smile like a kid and become more ready for the next time? The more we stop to recognise the way we perceive such moments affects the way we will record it in our brain. This is actively bringing about the growth mindset of Step 3.

As we move from starting something, where behaviours and patterns are fragile and new, we gain maturity that comes with progress and time in the form of growth. As you put in the effort, your level of familiarity and understanding becomes more directed and you are able to become more deliberate in your attention. The road to mastery is not always winning but recognising enough to be able to integrate your learnings into your wins, the true reward becoming seen in the form of maturity and growth. It is the insight you gain as you connect more deeply with your Athlete Within.

As we begin to recognise our mastery we can adjust our vision in different ways, look from different angles to better understand the gap that exists between our perception of what is and the expectations we hold. With this insight and clarity of the smaller details as well as the overarching, we can rehearse and recalibrate in a way that breaks down barriers and frees us from our own sense of limitations.

What are the signs? What is going to tell you that you are on your way, that there is progress and forward movement? Recognising is understanding your own dials, not just being goal focused but seeing the bits in between in the moments where life takes place. Your job is to recognise and link these connections with your own rituals and routines, your own why root, your own goals, your own mindset, and keep reminding yourself of the details of your Athlete Within that you set out along this path with in the beginning. In tweaking and working the dials you are constantly looking for improvements in the form of growth on the road to becoming your Athlete Within, all while being firmly planted in the vision of your future. With these helpful insights you develop maturity, mastery, and gain traction in other aspects of your life, creating a ripple effect in other areas of influence – everything aligns.

Exercise

Describe where you are today in rediscovering your Athlete Within. Does it feel the way you expected? Is this where you thought you would be?

Do you recognise the path you're taking and the steps you're making? How would you describe your Athlete Within to your mentor or coach?

Does rediscovering your Athlete Within excite your very being? Give details about your answer.

PAUSE TO ASSESS

We are all familiar with the rocky road of the middle years, recognising these are the years of change, the passage of time from the AM to the PM years of life, a new coming of age, a change in values, a change in perception of how we see the world. Often this passage is accompanied by events that give us a wake-up call, or a big jolt: a heart attack or cancer, financial struggles, a failed marriage or even a failed career. These are the big experiences, yet the 'roses' are the smaller and seemingly less obvious moments, the everyday joys that hold greater significance and meaning, the ones we really do need to stop and smell.

Pausing can be a simple ritual like journalling to capture the moments of meaning and magic. The actual act of writing in a journal takes us to a different part of our brain, to a different place where we become absorbed in our own world and spend time with ourselves. It could be like Julian, the lawyer, scheduling a weekly coffee meeting with the most important person in his world, himself. Pausing to assess is your own personal check in, to reflect, run through some questions and gauge your progress, your Athlete Within indicator.

Pausing to assess could be an external checkpoint too, a specific meet with your coach, mentor or accountability buddy to update and recalibrate. Pause to assess could be a window to refresh your proximity, the space you spend your time in. Even the simplicity of flowers can bring clarity and harmony to your space and more joy about who you are becoming as your Athlete Within.

Pausing to assess is a skill to be practised, and as you continue to refine and frequently check in, you become better at carving out time to evaluate, recognise and master.

Exercise

Have you planned a meeting with your Athlete Within to talk about your Athlete Within?

What are some of the wins, some of the losses, and what are you proud of so far?

CALIBRATE FORWARD

For your Athlete Within, calibrating forward is a step which takes you out of where you are now and into the future, projecting and considering what may be. Calibrating forward is stepping out of the moment. It gives you freedom to shake off all those rocks you are carrying around and see things in a different light, to perhaps rethink your strategy, and to more freely visualise and rehearse the way you are going about seeking your Athlete Within. This freedom can be a breath of fresh air, allowing you to let go of mistakes and failures, to see the new day in a new light, renew your energy and experience true progress.

Calibrating is clearing your head – you can then revisit your strategy, your direction, the structure you are following, the way your Athlete Within is unfolding. This gives the freedom to turn your attention to the factors leading up to the current scenario and looking at the future. Then metrics come into play. Working through your athletic profile, what are the expectations and perspectives on timing? Where should your focus be and what pace and feeling do you need to set? All of this is what brings in the precision, the quality and the ability to finish at your personal best.

Recognising is often about trusting your own process. You may not be able to see each and every step, yet you have calibrated forward so that you are clear on the direction of your Athlete Within.

Exercise

As you calibrate forward, what one thing did you let go of to experience freedom? Is this your ultimate upsetter?

What is working and what is not? What are the lessons or the insights for future reference? Where do you feel you should be spending more time to develop? What would you like to be moving away from?

This step is clearing the fog from the picture and getting in touch with your Athlete Within version of you. Looking for the gaps and what is coming at you.

10× THINKING

10× thinking is about shifting and stretching your path. It is stress testing your Athlete Within, designed not to make it bigger but to challenge you in your mind on how you see your vision and how to make it happen. If you run an event like a 42-kilometre marathon, it is a completely new event if you 10× it and think about it as a 420-kilometre run. What would you need to put in place then to achieve it?

In 10× thinking we are looking at the approach to our Athlete Within and ways that we can improve where we are as well as what we are doing. By shifting and stretching our design and image we have a new way of thinking: what else could we look at to develop our Athlete Within? Where could things get in our way? How could we be more resourceful, both internally such as mindset and externally with a coach or mentor? It is highlighting our application of our Athlete Within as well as being more deliberate in who we are becoming.

10× thinking is an interesting step of recognising progress as it takes you right into the unforeseen and the unpredictable, yet at the same time it can be quite revealing about what you are holding back. It could also be repeatedly asking a question ten times, taking you further into an answer than you have ever gone before. This is a crucial step, and is powerful when done in an environment that allows deep thought, continual answers (not hesitation) and repetition in gaining deeper understanding. With this in mind you can then adjust your deliberate attention.

Exercise

Why do you want to rediscover your Athlete Within? Keep repeating this same question ten times, looking for a deeper answer: what is behind your last answer, what is underneath, why do you believe that to be your truth? But why? But why?

> What would happen if you achieved your current goals 10× faster? Have you got the right mechanisms in place to not lose sight of your real dream of rediscovering your Athlete Within?

STEP UP

Stepping up is the analogy of stepping up to the plate. You come out of your bunker (your hiding hole) and out into the open, walk a few metres until you reach the plate, move your bat to a swinging action and then gaze at the pitcher, ready for the onslaught. It means leaving all your fears and ego back on the bench and stepping up. It is a place where you live in the moment, surrender yourself and trust that all you need is within you now.

All the practice and training has led up to this one moment. The speed of the ball is so fast in baseball that your hit begins even before the pitcher has let go of the ball. You commit.

You hear the word 'strike' from the referee behind you. Not a problem … I get three, right? You swing again, hearing the ball smack into the catcher's mitt behind you, and you already know before you hear the second strike. Step up and make this last one count. This time, you feel the pitcher, your eye is honed in, you swing your bat and you feel the connection. The ball heads high above first base and into the outfield. Without a moment's hesitation you are running, a hard sprint to land first base. 'Safe!' You made it.

We like predictability, we like control, we like to err towards safety, but we get excited when there's a good surprise. Stepping up is embracing whatever happens. It is an edge, a dance between the safe and the unknown. A dance between comfortable, giving it a go and taking a chance. It is realising you have the ability inside and now it is time to move faster and rise above the pack. To progress on your journey you need to step up. This is your time.

Often recognising also means change, finding the courage to move forward, make that decision, turning 'shoulds' into 'musts'. Stepping up is recognising our limitations, such as what decisions need to be made, what habits we need to tighten, and giving ourselves a time-frame and following through on our word.

Exercise

What is the thing you fear most about rediscovering your Athlete Within? Work on this to find the exact clarity and feeling and then discuss this with a mentor.

LEARNING FASTER

We all want to learn faster, but what is learning? Is it having more knowledge, filling our heads with more information like a thick textbook? Or is learning rather integrating the experiences we gain from life?

Every time we see something we stamp it with who we are in that moment. When you bring up a memory in your mind, you are actually reshaping it based on where you are and who you are at the time. Your brain is constantly making associations and integrating to keep you updated and relevant, bringing your best you to the equation.

Often a memory makes us feel a certain way, it takes us back to that past moment, we go back to that feeling. If this is a memory you enjoy, this can be a good thing. If it is an upsetting memory, you deepen the cut. Research shows we can be influenced by our proximity and create false memories, elaborating a story and bending the truth. How we 'see' our Athlete Within can be easily influenced if we let details slip. So how can we toughen up for the journey?

Federer was at the top of his game for more than two decades, and he has some secrets. One of these was to invite an up-and-coming wildcard player to his place to play. It increased the brotherhood of tennis, but it also provided Federer with a chance to sharpen his game. Playing a wildcard, the game was unpredictable. Think about it – a wildcard player is often younger, a little unpolished and full of hunger and excitement from playing the big name. They have nothing to lose. It intensified Federer's game, his instincts sharpened, he rose to the occasion, he learned faster.

Learning faster is putting yourself in situations which intensify your Athlete Within, build capacity and challenge you to become more, to create progress. Often it is following a thread, an opportunity to meet someone, share something, a feeling or challenge like a competition against a greater opponent. Learning faster is immersing yourself in greater experiences, where quality sleep meets deliberate skill and mindset, where a learning is accompanied by an intense emotion and activity. Learning faster is a form of studying. Our brains are plastic. Memories are made by connections of things that are associated. The more frequently you spend time recalling with deliberate clarity, the more you integrate and build your skillset. You could be honing learning faster into your Athlete Within with daily visualisation, disciplines or journaling using reflection.

Exercise

What could you do to challenge your Athlete Within to learn faster and progress?

Notes

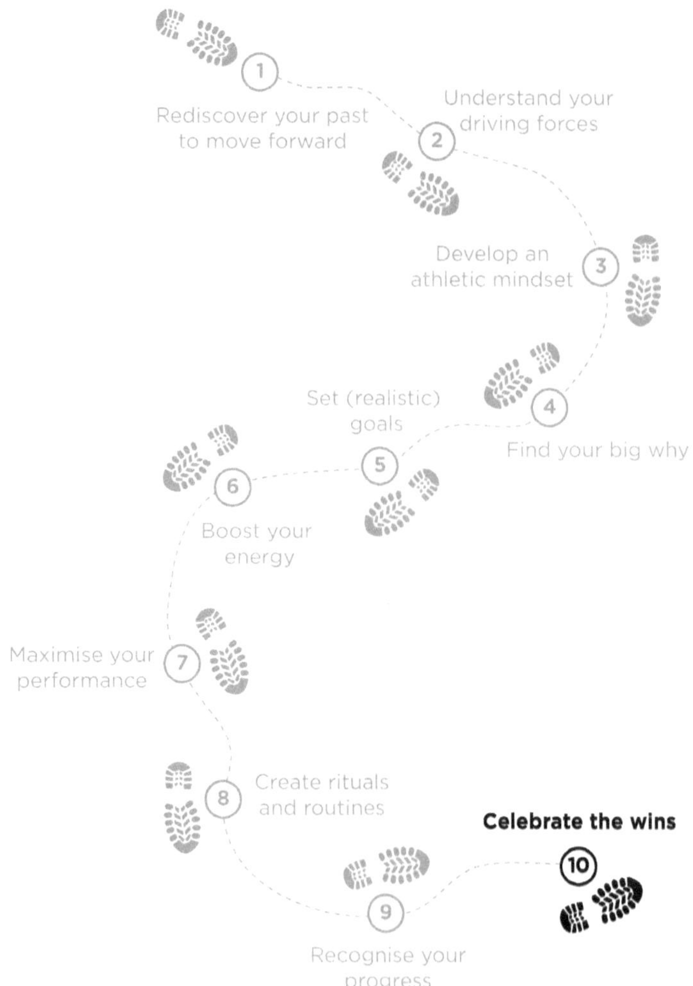

1
Rediscover your past to move forward
2
Understand your driving forces
3
Develop an athletic mindset
4
Find your big why
5
Set (realistic) goals
6
Boost your energy
7
Maximise your performance
8
Create rituals and routines
9
Recognise your progress
10
Celebrate the wins

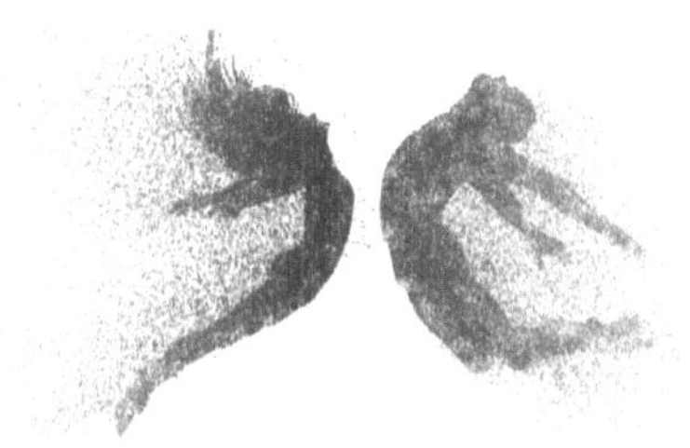

STEP 10:
CELEBRATE THE WINS

You are here! You've gone back to come forward. You have worked hard on yourself. You've come so far. There's one last thing that most of us are rubbish at but we cannot forget to do as it's an essential part of your Athlete Within: embrace gratitude and celebrate. Realising you're in a beautiful place, right now, the dots are connecting. Welcome home, a place you have looked for, dreamt about and are now reaching.

When was the last time you celebrated something about your own life that is not a birthday? Why is it we tend to hold a stigma attached to taking time out, stopping to celebrate a win and share a moment?

The way we celebrate is about more than acknowledgment, it is part of our self-talk, part of a winning mentality. For the Athlete Within, it is a way of seeing the world. It encourages growth, more experimentation and further exploration. Take the time to breathe in the moment, feeling the connection with the experience. It's your chance to feel more alive in that moment. It is recognition that fires up good emotions inside your body and feeds your very soul. It builds momentum. It builds a can-do attitude that leaves you thirsty for more. I'll be back tomorrow to do this again and add some more. For a kid, this is all part of a normal day of play. For an adult it is learning to be playful, to be on the lookout for things to celebrate, to create a readiness that sets the tone for every day.

A celebration is a reminder you are moving in the right direction, your reward. It means stepping slightly out of the moment to observe, feel and capture the moment – your own mental photo. The celebration is then you putting your stamp on it. Defining it as your moment and giving yourself the gift of enjoying it, a little clap of celebration and you whisper 'winning'.

Do you really need a reason to celebrate? Do you need a reminder? A date? Be proactive. Be your playful self. Maybe bring in some heart, some gratitude, smile and allow yourself your moment.

Every elite athlete looks forward to receiving a medal, a trophy, a ribbon. But behind every celebration there is a story where the real wins were already being made, one step after the other. Every athlete is a winner before they walk to the starting line, just for showing up and participating. That's the real story behind the win.

Tim was early 30s, newly married and halfway through his wife's first pregnancy. All a bit of a dream really, yet to him life felt like going up a very steep hill. His conversations were changing and he had a new favourite phrase, 'the inevitable' – the unavoidable truth no one talks about. One day he was particularly perky after a visit to the obstetrician, greeting me with a handshake and the words, 'Hi, I'm the chequebook'. I'm the guy, the third wheel, the one always a step behind, I don't have the shiny ring and I'm not the one carrying the baby.

Of course Tim could see how the story played, it's just he seemed to pick up the wrong script. He just needed some editing. I asked him if he was a fun guy; of course he said yes. 'So when was the last time you were a fun guy?' I asked. He went quiet, he went dark, he went within. 'I'm not sure,' he said.

He started to talk and he became swamped with overwhelm: 'How are we going to get together a deposit, buy a house, and get through all the hurdles?' In some ways he was frustrated no one had told him how it would play out. I asked Tim how much he needed. He looked confused. I said, 'Well, you have clearly put a lot of thought into the cost of all these things, so how much do you need? What's the cost for the next five years?' Of course he didn't have any answers. He was just stuck in a thought train and didn't know where he was getting off.

'Let's play ball,' I said. 'Let's say everything goes exactly as planned … where will you be in seven years?' No reply, as there was no answer. He barely knew what was happening after their baby's birth.

'What if I was sitting on a verandah, looking out over the ocean with the waves coming in and you were telling me how the last seven years actually panned out?' He took the challenge. I organised a coffee catch-up and two weeks later I went to meet him for his answer.

He described how the question really disturbed him. It stayed in his mind for days. Then he spoke to his wife about it, asking her the same question. To his surprise she had a clear answer. Talking gave him words to help describe how he was feeling, to see his roadblocks, and how to overcome them. He wanted to become more fun. He wanted to connect more. He wanted to be more than just 'a wallet'. He spoke to me for almost an hour and at the end I asked him: 'How are you going to remind yourself about this conversation so you don't fall back into your old you?'

He smiled then he laughed: 'This morning, as I was putting my shoes on to come see you, I was thinking exactly that. Then I wondered at what age do kids learn to tie their shoe laces and it came to me.'

Every morning as I tie my shoes is my one minute to connect and celebrate the person I am and the person I am becoming.'

One aspect of inspiring your Athlete Within is developing key habits that nourish your heart and soul. Celebration is knowing 'how to' celebrate. It is turning it into a part of that winning mindset, living at the level of growth. It takes you to a new place, developing an open mind, seeing and noticing when moments happen. It is when these moments are taking place with increasing repetition that you know you are on the right track and moving in the right direction.

Celebration is also sharing, because your achievements hold an even bigger meaning when you celebrate them with people who hold a special place in your life. It is putting down the competition for a moment and coming together because sharing is what unites us. It's the glue that brings us together and lifts our energy, ready for the next step.

RECOGNISE AND EMBRACE THE MOMENTS

Moments slide by. The kids seem to grow up so quickly. Suddenly it feels like yesterday you were in your 30s then today you're well into your 50s. How often do you stop to laugh, to savour the seasons' change, to notice someone is wearing new shoes? Recognising is more than just noticing, it is living with a sense of excitement and anticipation that life is always happening. It is being in the right space to recognise.

At first it feels like an effort, having to recognise things that are changing or things that are new around us. This rings true especially because many of us are not used to seeing the wins, the golden moments, and we take them for granted or we don't consider them worthy enough for a celebration. But then, with practice, it feels like you are building a new habit, and you are. It is continually working till it becomes a part of you, another dimension in how you see the world.

When we sit at the table for dinner, our six-year-old twins always ask: 'What was your favourite thing today?' It's become a routine, one that we love. It pushes us to stop for a moment, take a deep breath and scout through the memories of the day for what was special, even magical, worthy of mention. Some days 'nothing' happens. Get up, eat, go to work, pick up the kids, cook, eat, go to bed. The thing is, we can still find something to cherish even in the most normal of days, the routine. For the twins, it is often playing on the monkey bars or pasta in their lunchbox. For me, it's a coffee break with Lisa or a run with my son. The secret is training the mind to connect to the heart so we can see it all.

A life of meaning is recognising the details in your life.

I find we are often harder on ourselves than we realise, setting a bar that may not be realistic and may not be relevant to who we are in this moment. It may be time to reset the clocks, to work on our growth mindset and go searching and hunt for personal moments. Moments that reflect where you are at, what you are thinking about, what has meaning only to you.

Exercise

Take some videos and photos, pop them in a digital frame and add music to it. Use this story to help you recognise moments. Go back to it. It's a powerful tool to help you bring attention to what matters to you and to the now. It's an important step to include in your celebrations.

What else can you do to help you recognise the moments?

Once you start to recognise the moments that make your life special and give it meaning, how do you embrace them? Are you an 'in the moment' kind of person, a quick internal 'pat on the back' then that's all and back to the grind? Or maybe you erect the wall of fame, one of those houses where you walk in to an entrance filled with trophies, family photos and reminders? Or do you let the moments pass by, not really speaking up, jumping up, just a quiet thought, then you file them away?

It's clear that even in the way we embrace the moments, we are all individual and have our own ways of doing it. And that's okay. The most important thing is to grab those moments and make them special, significant milestones that will form part of who you are in a meaningful way.

We all have a story, either our own or one close enough to cause a shift. Embracing the moments has a greater meaning personally since my own walk down the road of cancer. I have a very strong feeling of living my second stage of life, being fully aware of the stats and the context of who I was being. Often the big moments cause us to embrace the small moments. For me, coming out of cancer, I see the world in a different way.

Embracing moments is about the relationship you have with yourself. Things may not always be moving to plan or the way you expected. By embracing the moment you can step back and see it for what it is: a part of life. The significance may not always be clear in the moment but taking the experience with you could be a part of your growing and learning how to attach and detach. Maybe seeing the lesson or taking it on board is akin to the apprentice on the path towards mastery, and the wisdom is growing within.

Embracing moments is a very personal thing. There are no instructions. It is more heart, more in the now, what feels right to you. My biggest encouragement to you is turn the volume up and embrace the moments, whether that be for yourself or celebrating someone else.

Exercise

How do you like to embrace moments? Do you like to capture them in a way you can return to? Or do you like to enjoy the moment for what it is and then let it go?

A LIFE WELL LIVED

What makes a life well lived? Fast and furious, like striking a match? Full of adventure, taking the world by storm? Or quietly living out a long life in the old ways? The spectrum is broad, the peaks and troughs can be many, like the waves on a beach or the ripples of a lake. With a bit of thought, you may answer that a life well lived comes back to finding meaning and purpose so that your time here has substance. Like an onion, it has layers of productivity and achievement, measurable outcomes towards the outside, then as you dig deeper you get closer and closer to the essence.

So far in this step we have focused on the importance of celebration. Moments of importance like a win, taking the time to recognise moments as windows deeper into who we are, embracing these as steps in the right direction and maximising them so we can create more. A path forward as we learn on the way of life.

But what is a life well lived?

When we grow, we collect a lot of expectations of how we should live and the way we should be, yet rarely do we stop to decide for ourselves what it means to us to be fulfilled, to live a life we are happy about and proud of. And on top of this, as we experience more and gain wisdom, this idea of a well-lived life is shaped by our external environment as well as our own feelings.

My own life was the perfect example of all this.

Physically, I would go in and out of training, finishing a winter and arriving at summer only to be driven to develop my athlete by my shape and aesthetics. It was a stop–start mentality dictated by what I saw on the outside, a far cry from the slow burn philosophy required to discover the Athlete Within. Emotionally I was on a roller-coaster too. On one hand a looming divorce meant my days were filled with conflict and apathy. On the other the sadness I was experiencing pushed me to take a serious look at myself and pull that grand old question out again: 'Is this a life well lived?'

It was a chaotic push and pull both internally and externally. Then it dawned on me. To define what a life well lived is, I had to approach it from every angle. And that's what I'm asking you to do right here.

Find an overarching vision of what life means to you and the direction you want to head. It is about setting an expectation of your future. This expectation of the future has to match who you are today. What are you doing today? Who are you being that fulfils your vision? Are you living towards your vision, becoming congruent with who you are and who you are becoming?

You can think about your life well lived but you also need to experience it, feel it: you have to put your body on the line, add your physical self to the mix. Are you doing what is congruent for your body? Are you following your internal blueprint and moving enough?

For me a life well lived is about uncovering more of your essence on a path of becoming and growing. Growth is about overcoming, embracing your existence and finding your own sense of self, your own freedom. And realising you are unable to control your environment, you can only control your sense of you, so let life unfold. Rediscovering your Athlete Within is a process, finding your own way to live that is congruent to your individuality and leaving you smiling with gratitude.

Notes

—

PART III

WHO **YOU** WILL **BECOME**

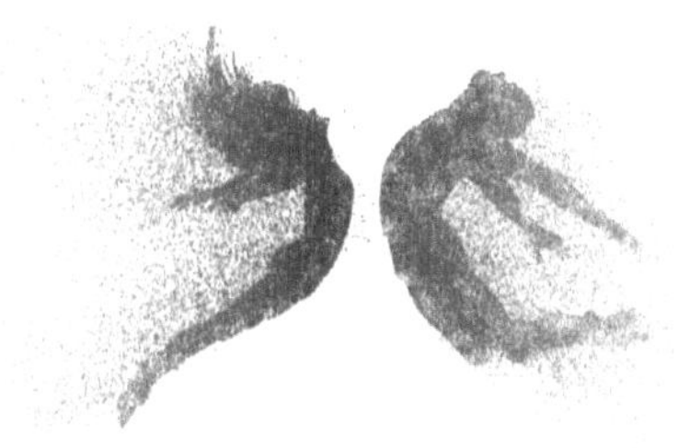

SO HOW ABOUT JANE?

'I did it! I finished the walk!' Those were Jane's words when she opened the door.

Yes. She did finish her walk. And through it all she had to flip her life, start believing in herself and rewrite her future … her way.

She dived deep into her past to rediscover what brought her joy. She smiled, she cried, she felt the hopes and crashes of her past years. The failures, the wins, the missed opportunities, the achievements.

She reviewed her beliefs and embraced change, stepping out of her usual patterns humbly trying new things.

She worked on her mindset and focused on grit and grind to grow. She tackled her ultimate upsetter and changed her habits one at a time, slowly, with intention. She enlisted the help of her friends to keep her accountable and formed her A team.

She found purpose in being active to help others and as a result started helping herself. She got unstuck and moved forward.

She set goals and checkpoints, rituals and routines, and ticked them all off, sometimes with ease sometimes with blood, sweat and tears. But she felt energy growing with each step and she had something bigger now inside driving her on.

She stuck to her program in and out of the clinic, she primed her body, building stability and strength, working her breath and performance out and about, in the biological gym, chatting away with her friends.

She stopped at every opportunity to assess her progress. She knew she was getting stronger, happier, more and more ready to go on that bloody long walk, and savouring the little wins made her sure about the path ahead. She could see it, she could feel it, she was living it. And she often celebrated, with her friends, with herself, because every moment added up to the big ones. She became her Athlete Within.

Every year Jane and her friends walk the long walk and every year they raise a crazy amount of money for charity. It has become part of their identity. In between, during the other 364 days of the year, Jane lives through the ripple effects that her journey of rediscovery have brought her.

Jane walks most days, not because she's training for her walk, but because that's what brings her joy, energy, feeds her big why and fills her soul. Walking is just part of who she now is and it is second nature to her, just like sleeping or breathing. Some days she goes for hours, some just for mere minutes. When her body needs a break she recoups her strength by slowing down, pulling weeds in her backyard, pruning the roses, stopping to have a cup of tea under the shade of a big tree. And when it rains she puts on a raincoat and still goes outside or crawls up on the sofa for a little meditation, working on her breathing, her mindfulness. She makes time for her children. She makes time for her new husband. She makes time for herself.

Just like everyone else, Jane has her ups and downs, moments when she is challenged and life pulls her in different directions. In those moments she brings it back to the core, the simplest thing for her to do: walk. Chaos is still around but there is no storm inside. Her why is steering her forward, steady, clear, confident in the path ahead.

Her life now has quality, she's ready for her PM and for all the possibilities.

Jane has become who she was destined to be from the day her little Athlete Within was born.

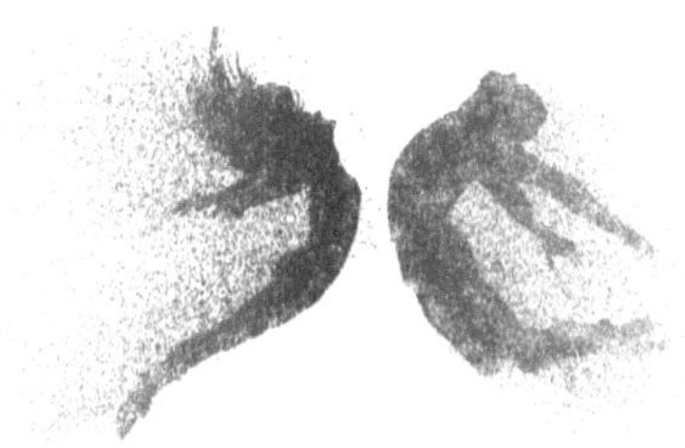

BE YOU

There is a tradition in our house: every year we sit down to watch *Love Actually*. It's a family event, decked out with an inside picnic with our Christmas tree in the background. It is then my role to ask the dad questions like, 'Haven't we watched this already?' 'Have the characters grown older over the past year?', (spoiler alert) 'Is Sarah finally going out with Karl?' – until my son, now 15, brings the laughter. My wife takes all these comments in her stride because it sets the feeling for Christmas, the ending of another year, and if you look around 'it seems to me that love, actually, is everywhere'. Sorry …

That's one of my highlights of the year, every year.

What does life mean to you? What are your highlights? And where to from here?

Making real change is never easy – that is understood. The door to a new chapter is heavy, the lock and combination has its own complexity, with rust on the hinges formed through time. Yet with patience, you bring more of you out. You find a way. Your version of the movie you are watching is yours to hold onto, to share, to then become part of something bigger, to matter. What we talk about we bring about, what we think we create, what we share grows and who we are shines brighter. Bottling up is a strategy towards tragedy. Remember? As author Wayne Dyer wrote, don't die with your music still inside.

Rediscovering your Athlete Within is in many ways a process to draw out what already exists within you, to awaken a part of you that may have been buried as life just happened.

Often we try to turn dreams into success and achievements, targets which carry inherent pressures. As you move through these cycles you head towards more of you. You know when you are living more of you because the pressures and strains are not seen as difficult but rather more as excitement, even moments to celebrate. You have changed your perspective and you are in tune with who you are. When we find this congruency we are uplifted naturally by its pull. We wake up feeling compelled, wanting to live more fully in this life. It is your individuality, your uniqueness you bring to the world. You shine.

Author Andrew Griffiths tells a story of a friend who gets stressed every time she walks up on stage to speak – and she is a speaker. Her heart rate goes up, she feels sick in the stomach like there is a heat taking over her whole body. He then describes an interview he saw of Bruce Springsteen just before he walked out on stage, telling the interviewer he is just so excited and pumped to get up in front of the audience, because his heart rate is up, he is feeling sick and his body is feeling flushed. It's perception. It's who we are and how we approach life. It's our own way.

Authenticity is a risk. You're going somewhere you haven't been before and meeting that part of you, that energy, that personal expression.

Authenticity requires you to be more you than you even knew was there before.

Authenticity requires giving words to your unique spark, your ideas and your perspectives.

Authenticity requires putting a part of you into form and expression. It is revealing, exposing, vulnerable, open.

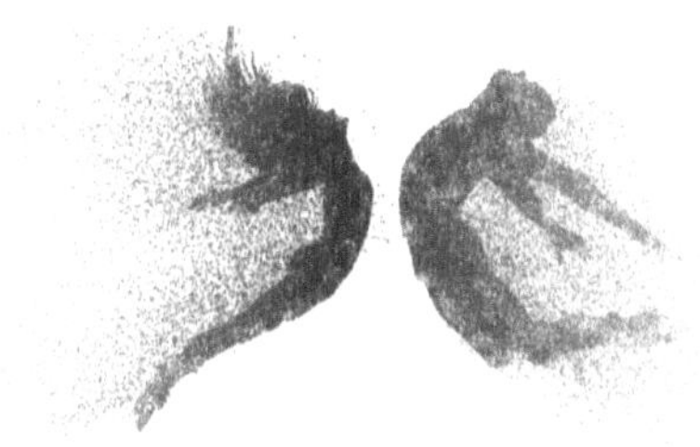

BECOME THE MASTER

Inside each of us is a master. We began our journey as a clumsy apprentice with a heart full of hope that at times fell in puddles, at times climbed mountains. We followed the course of our meandering river, often making a good run and just as often crashing over the falls.

It was our ancestors who forged a new path, stepping out onto the savannah, learning to think on their feet and develop advantages that would help us adapt to almost every environment on Earth, and one day, beyond. One such ability is in the mind, to develop insight, to forward plan and calibrate interaction, to build expectations as well as the courage to search for freedom and, above all, the ability of wonder and curiosity that feeds our creativity.

The journey for the Athlete Within is not a straight one. On the surface, its principles are fundamental to our blueprint, but as we move deeper, it challenges the very way we live. As with all things, rarely is there a recipe to live by. The teacher's greatest gift is to guide. The Athlete Within knows the truth lies in becoming the eternal student of life. As the river unfolds, we begin to understand that becoming is not stopping the river, trying to control or dam the waters or even intercept them, but the process of allowing. It is when the human is 'being' that we realise the best place to sit for the allowing is up high on the hill, where the grass is green, the harvest is plenty and the view is grand.

EPILOGUE

When I was 10 years old my parents took our family on a (rather long) coach trip to the red deserts of Central Australia. Each late afternoon when the coach stopped, we set up our camp kitchen and single pole tents, bathed in the light of the wide desert sunset. In the morning we were up before sunrise, reversing the previous night's order: dismantling the tents, packing up the kitchen, putting everything in the belly of the coach. Being young, my brother and I were not at all interested in this daily chore and got bored before the day even begun.

One morning, the driver, recognising our growing mischief, sent us ahead and we walked up to a small group of people who had also left the camp on foot to give others time to sort out their belongings and pack the coach. Some were walking while others decided to move off at a slow jog, taking in the early morning light, the red desert that stretched out with its wide horizon.

The following day we did exactly the same, and it was clear a morning ritual had started to form. People would leave camp before the coach and stretch out on the two-lane highway at their own pace, lost in their own worlds.

One particularly early morning I tagged on to the running group, joining in with conversations that quickly turned into silence, the surroundings too powerful a voice to allow us to use any word. Without realising, I soon left the group behind, driven by a stride that felt right, running like I could go for days. I was in my own lane, in my own space.

I didn't even hear the coach closely approaching, the driver indicating his presence with a light sound of the horn. I pulled over and waited for the coach to stop. As the door glided open, the driver turned to me with a big smile, laughing: 'I was starting to think I had missed you, you have run so far this morning.' Jumping up the three stairs to get to my seat, I was met by loud applause, congratulations and high-fives walking down the aisle. The song was burned into my mind: the Australian desert etched in my memory, the flavour of success, the feeling in my body forever with me.

A year ago, when we first moved to Tasmania and into our rental at the foot of a very steep hill, I vividly remember looking up and feeling a strong pull, a longing, a wish to tackle the mountain and just run. Not long after, one late afternoon, I put on my shoes and went for a walk, up the bush trail and to the end of the reserve. Feeling my feet on the terrain I quickly got lost in my own space, my own time, and I was running. Without realising I reached the top. I turned around, looked down at Hobart and I instantly knew my being up there wasn't the result of a specific decision I had made, I was more following an urge, something I desired deep inside.

Then the sky started to turn a light pink and I could anticipate the first signs of a sunset. The beat inside of me started to surface, my desert song playing louder and louder. The memory of that holiday flashed before my eyes and I was there, reliving a moment of true happiness. You know, one of those instants that cannot really be repeated, just savoured and embraced for their simplicity, their rawness, their completeness.

I wasn't 10 years old anymore, I was 52. A life well lived (so far), dreams for my future and love in my life. I knew there and then that the years ahead of me would be the best ones yet.

ACKNOWLEDGMENTS

There are many amazing people who have contributed to writing *Rediscover Your Athlete Within*.

If it weren't for the encouragement of Andrew Griffiths – incredible mentor and now friend, a man who is patient beyond measure, humble yet strong – this book would never have made the light of day. Thank you for supporting me all the way through and for believing in me.

Thank you to my editor Michael Hanrahan and his team at Publish Central, for guiding me through the writing process and answering all my questions with your trademark professional, calm, easy-to-deal-with attitude and forever smiling face. My incredible accountability buddies: Bronwyn Reid, Ally Muller, Lalita Lowe – thank you for the endless hours on the phone and your spurring me on. Julia Kuris, your cover is just lit! You rock.

I got to this exciting point in my life because of all the amazing people I've met through the years who have left an indelible mark and have helped shape who I am today. They are my life tribe. You are too many to even begin.

My shining star is my wife Lisa, for grounding me when my creativity flows (a bit too much), surprising me when life seems ordinary, for helping shape and challenge every single idea in this book and encouraging me to be more of who I am in her own unique way. Your love and unwavering commitment to us are the constant in my life I never take for granted. Thank you for teaching me grammar and for reminding me to buy you flowers.

Thank you Mum and Dad for choosing to live on the edge of the bush, my beloved playground. To my brother Stephen for endless hours playing, imagining and exploring. Fast forward to now – I cherish your opinion for your straight up, down the line version of how the world works. To my best friend Jason, for the hours spent playing *anything*, often with some kind of ball involved to the sounds of Boom Crash Opera.

And a heartfelt THANK YOU…

To Larry Markson: The Cabin Experience changed me.

To my mentors and outright legends, Dr John Kelly, Dr Stephen Esposito, Dr Wayne Minter, Dr Doug Herron, Dr Clinton McCauley, Dr Laurence Tham.

To Professor Pavel Kolar, for sharing his passion over the years and making me fall in love with DNS.

To Professor Alena Kobesova, Petra Valouchová, Marcela Safarova and Martina Ježková, for going above and beyond teaching the wonders of DNS.

To Dr Michael and Maggie Rintala, for pushing the boundaries of what's possible.

To the incredible professionals who inhabit the world of TMJ, sleep and chronic pain: Dr Charlotte de Courcey-Bayley, Dr Karen McCloy, Dr Steven Olmos, Dr Mayoor Patel, Catherine Norton, for your guidance and inspiration.

To Megumi Bennet, my bonsai Master, for teaching me that to understand the tree is to understand life. To Graeme Clark, my classical guitar teacher, for pushing me to see performance in a completely different light.

To the many clients I have had the pleasure to work with over the years, the relationship is always two ways – as you learn so do I.

As with all things, some pushed my buttons more, test me further, they raised the bar and I had to grow to meet them there. Sophie Woods, Charlotte van Veenendaal, the Wrights, the Klingers, the McLellands, Nathan Hepple and Sarah Tempest, Jenny Josling, Jill Fulcher, Chris Lavelle.

To my Chiro tribe, for being my forever sounding board, Drs: Murray Warner, Kim Lie Jom, Ravi Rudner, Kara Hayes, Tom Waller, Peter Geroulas, Petros Vournelis, Andrea Sergeant.

To old and new friends, for being your amazing you: Anna Calvert, Simon Dawe, Chris Orfanos, Aaron James, Craig Wilson, Lorraine Khouri, Sue Templeman, Kirby Wright.

To Craig Anderson for shaping my ultimate vision of the Athlete Within – you are it.

ABOUT THE AUTHORS

Dr Brett Lillie grew up at the edge of the bush in the northern suburbs of Sydney, Australia. From the moment he could walk, his legs would instinctively take him right into the outdoors, where he started growing a deep love and connection to the land and everything physical. Skateboarding down the steep driveway, building forts with his best friends, jumping in the ocean on hot summer days, exploring the bush. He could not be stopped: he had to go, and get there fast.

Sharing the surname Lillie with one of Australia's cricket greats (and no, he is not related) inevitably meant that a ball and a bat were a large part of his games growing up. His memories of late afternoons spent with his grandfather throwing and catching a ball still resonate strongly today and form the roots of his very own Athlete Within.

His innate desire to be active and study anything related to human movement is definitely one of the many factors that threw Dr Brett into the world of rehabilitation. A zoology degree quickly turned into a Master in Chiropractic and Dr Brett set up his own clinic in the heart of the city. Through the years practising, he never stopped learning, pushing himself to grow and be open to change. His uncanny ability to be drawn towards visionaries who push boundaries in their own fields, whatever part of the world they reside, made Dr Brett travel across many oceans to study from the best in rehab, dentistry, sleep and chronic pain. A cross pollination that spans across many disciplines, his true love being movement.

Then life happened. A divorce, a serious illness, deep family loss and the feeling that surely there was more to life than just stress and struggle. He embarked on a journey of self-exploration and deep change, one that saw him question many things of the past and take hold of his future.

It was after a serendipitous conversation with Professor Stuart McGill – the BackFitPro – who candidly admitted being fitter at 78 than when he was 50, that the idea of *Rediscover Your Athlete Within* was born. The rest, as they say, is history, and the journey continues.

Everyone who's met Dr Brett has been touched in one way or another by his free spirit, his deep knowledge, his caring heart, love of life and contagious laughter. Today, he lives in Tasmania with his family, in a house on the side of a mountain. And when he's not helping someone rediscover their Athlete Within, you can find him running up and down the hills of Hobart, taking in life and the magical view.

Lisa Lillie was born in the Italian part of Switzerland, where lakes meet mountains and snow drops at sea level. She learnt to ski before the training wheels came off her bike; her summers were spent hiking with the family, being outside with her cousin Linda and her friends, always on the hunt for adventure. She loved ice hockey, watching the Tour de France with her nonno and playing tennis. Karate was her one true love.

Lisa played the organ, guitar and loved singing. She excelled at languages (let's not talk Latin) and anything requiring an artistic flare. The important women in her life were all excellent cooks. They nurtured her interest in food and made sure there was always something fresh and smelling delicious on the table, ready to share with everyone. Growing up in a tight-knit community, with roots planted deep, allowed her to feed her curiosity and venture far and wide until she reached Australia…and she felt right at home.

Dotted along the line you can see the seeds that grew into who Lisa is today. In between the business of running a family and working alongside Dr Brett, she makes time to hike, explore the outdoors and is now back in the dojo doing Karate. Her inner athlete, she muses, is definitely a chef and the kitchen is her gym. Kneading fresh bread is her arm day, making a roast is her leg day and foraging along the streets of Hobart is her cardio.

Lisa has definitely gone full circle. Having moved to the Switzerland of the Southern Hemisphere, she loves the quieter lifestyle, one that reminds her very much of her childhood. If she's not in the kitchen cooking up a storm you can find her in the garden pruning the hedge or her favourite rose bushes.

Don't be fooled by Lisa's want to be in the background of *Rediscover Your Athlete Within*. She has contributed to this book in every step and every aspect and her voice shines through in every page. Her knowledge born from working in the clinic with Dr Brett and her own search for the Athlete Within has brought a freshness and relatability for the reader to enjoy.

SHARE YOUR STORY

Every time I hear someone telling me their story of rediscovery, well… my heart literally jumps. I am instantly inspired to keep improving, keep going, to work on my own athlete within, and the burning desire I have to be at the service of others increases tenfold. That's because we all play a part in helping each other be our best.

I would love to hear from you. I would love to hear YOUR story. What did you discover, who's your Athlete Within? What is your big why? Have you allowed yourself to dream? What was your biggest challenge, what did you have to overcome?

Your story can help others find their way back and take their first steps towards their new future.

Share your story - email me at **hello@brettlillie.com**

WELL HELLO THERE ATHLETE WITHIN

How did you go?
Did you enjoy the book?

I'd love it if you could leave a review on your favourite e-store and **help me help others** rediscover their Athlete Within.

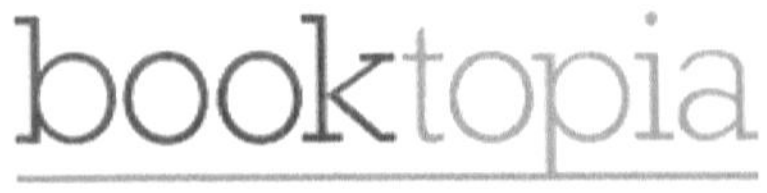
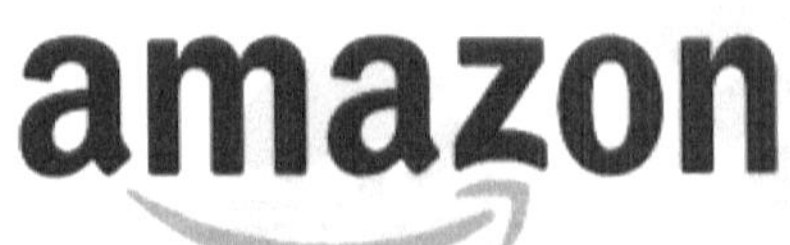

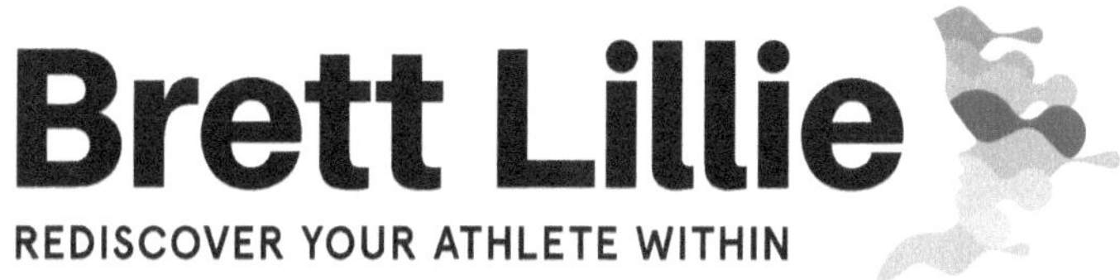

Are you ready to Rediscover your athlete within?

If you've been inspired by Dr Brett's book, there are a number of ways you can now work with him and kickstart your journey of rediscovery.

Keep reading the information on the following pages or visit his website at **www.brettlillie.com** for all the details. You can also join his great community on Facebook, LinkedIn and Instagram.

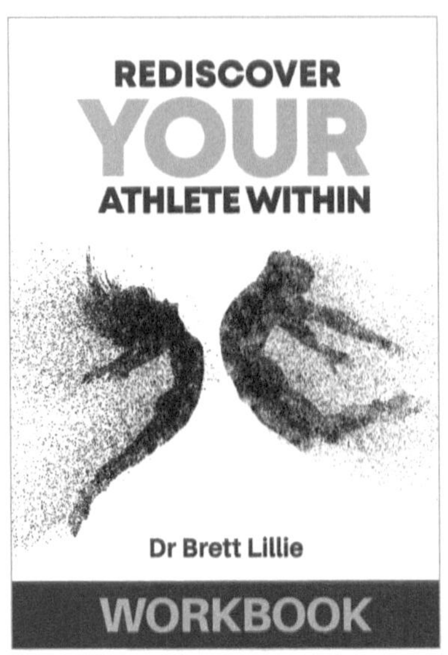

Download your free *Rediscover Your Athlete Within* Workbook

One of the best and most effective strategies to help you rediscover your Athlete Within is to WRITE. Doodles, lists, words, ideas, diagrams, quotes, feelings, thoughts...when you put them on paper they instantly come to life and they can help you materialise your dream life a lot clearer, a lot stronger, a lot faster.

To support your journey of rediscovery, I have designed a workbook that mirrors the 10-step process of this book. Inside you'll find all the exercises you've just been reading about and some fun surprises to keep you motivated and on track.

Hop over to my website **brettlillie.com** to download your free copy of *Rediscover Your Athlete Within* workbook.

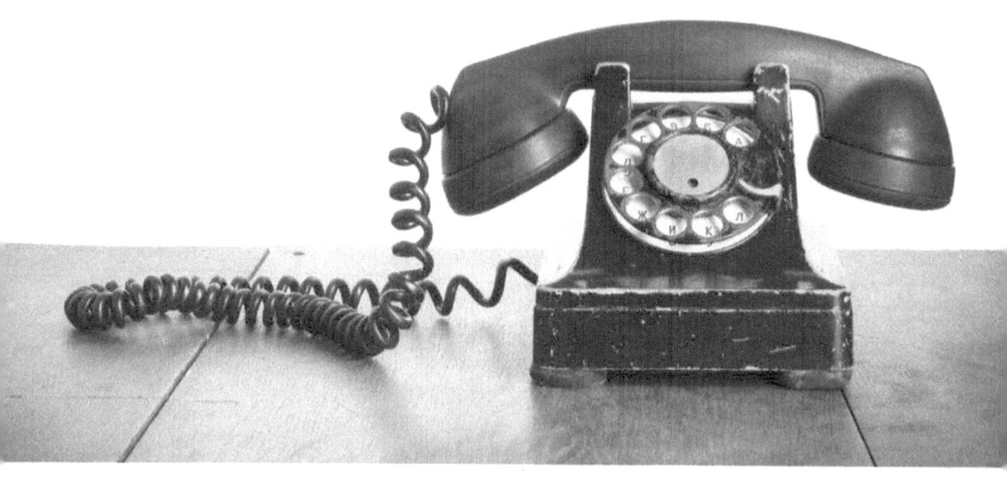

An athletic match made in heaven

You're ready to rediscover your athlete within and want to work with the best. However, the best sometimes is not the best for YOU. Like in any relationship, you can only achieve great results with people who are willing to work as hard as you and support you through it all.

Let's see if you and Dr Brett are a great match and can form your dream team.

Book a complimentary focus call with Dr Brett to discuss the best way to work together. During the session you'll be able to share your concerns, doubts, hopes and dreams and ask Dr Brett questions about how he can help and support your inner athlete while you embark on this new journey of rediscovery.

Get in touch with Dr Brett's team at **hello@brettlillie.com** to book a call. They will email you some prelim questions so you can be sure to make the most out of your time.

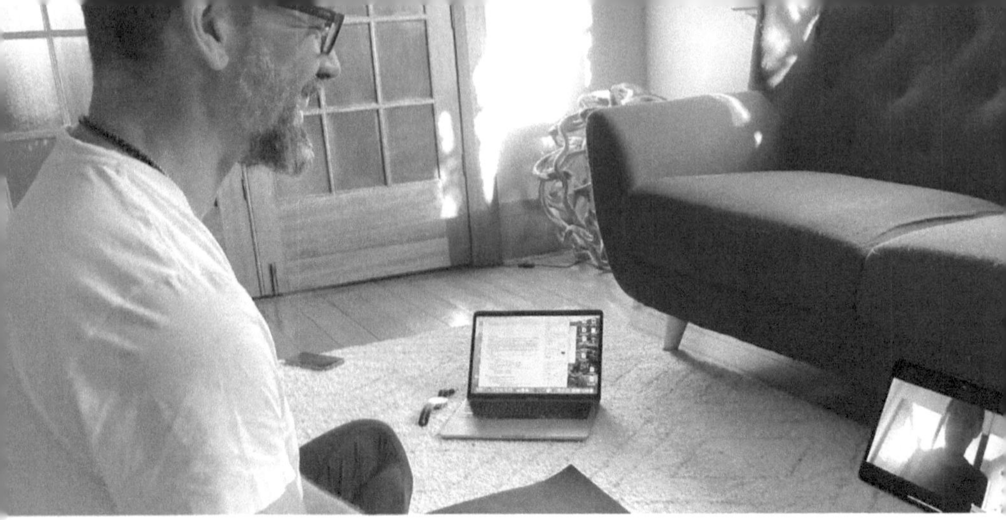

Would you like to work 1:1 with Dr Brett

You know you have everything inside of you to rediscover your athlete within but starting can be hard and staying on the path even harder. Old habits pull you in creating confusion and fuelling procrastination.

Dr Brett works with people from all walks of life to cut through the noise and help them get off the couch and get moving again. Some may need a little nudge others a big kick, but everyone working with him will be guided with knowledge care and just the right amount of toughness so they can be certain to park the doubts and create a shift for the better.

Dr Brett's focus is on creating clarity, inspiration and support for all his inner athletes. One message you would have taken away from this book is that living a active lifestyle is the key to longevity and the time to be active is now.

If you'd like to find out more about working with
Brett please email hello@brettlillie.com

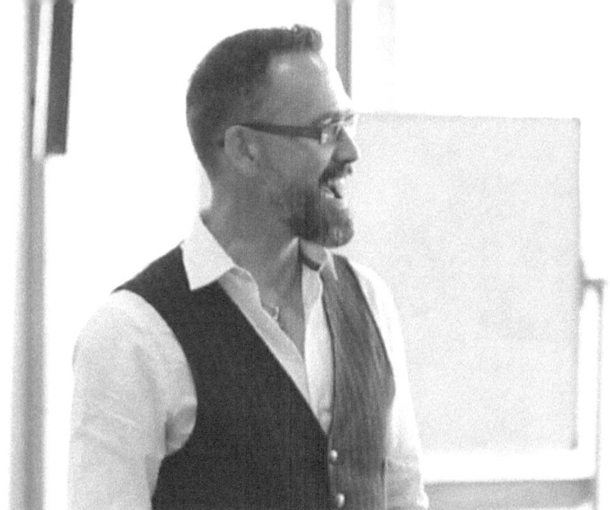

If you think this book is the bee's knees, wait till you see the workshops

Dr Brett's workshops are the perfect starting point to help you rediscover your athlete within and form a clear path forward to enjoy an active lifestyle.

Set In small and informal settings, these workshops are all about supporting you to uncover and further develop your athletic abilities. You'll learn more about your mindset and explore what you're capable of. You will walk away with practical strategies, frameworks and even hands-on exercises you can apply to your every day. Dr Brett will make you think on your feet (literally) and inspire you to continue your journey of rediscovery.

If you'd like to know more about joining one of Dr Brett's workshops, check out the details and the upcoming dates at www.brettlillie.com.

Spaces are limited.

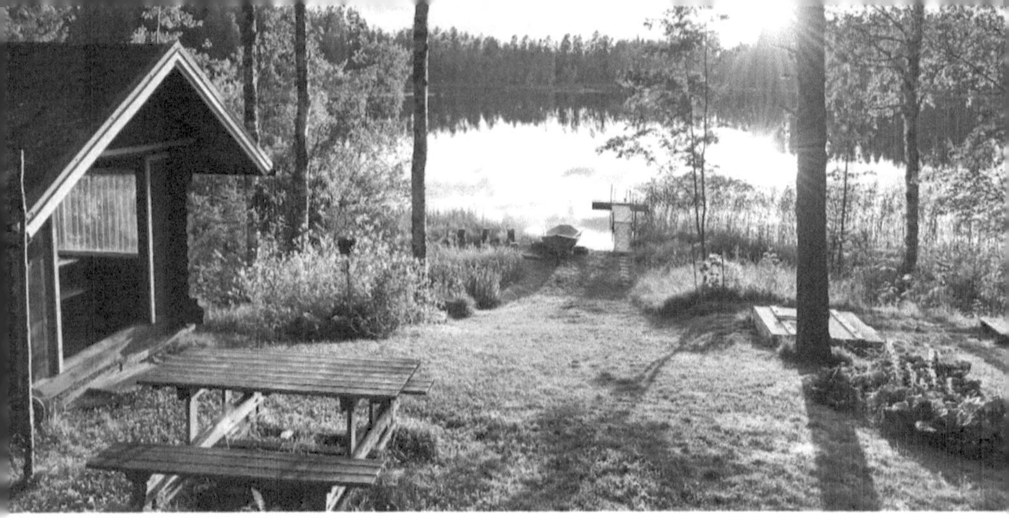

A transformative experience to discover and become your athlete within

This is an exclusive 4 day retreat designed for people who are ready to go after their dream lives. Run in a relaxed setting, away from daily distractions and routines, this program is a full immersion in all things athlete within.

Dr Brett will guide you through targeted activities to challenge your beliefs and help you embrace those parts of your life that need a shake up. He will teach you how to train your mindset like an athlete, increase your energy levels, discover what drives you to keep going and show you how to exercise smarter not harder.

Dr Brett's biggest wish for everyone attending this retreat is to walk away having uncovered their inner athlete, confident in their path ahead. To do so he will share simple, practical and effective tools to help everyone progress even after they're thrusted back into their busy lives.

If you're interested in joining Dr Brett's exclusive retreat, please contact his staff on hello@brettlillie.com.

More information is available on www.brettlillie.com

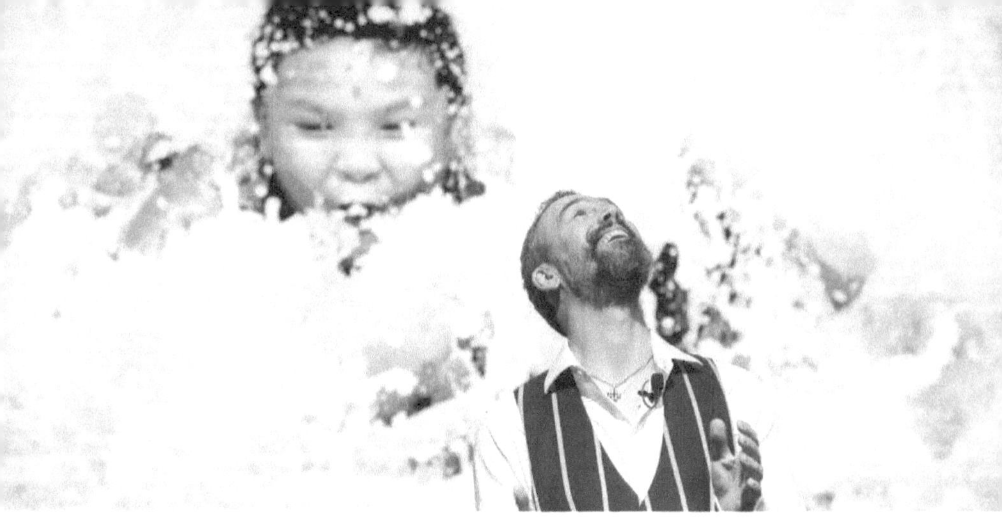

Want to inspire your audience with an engaging, experienced and energetic speaker?

Dr Brett is a dynamic, thoughtful and skilful speaker who's been presenting to live and virtual audiences in Australia and beyond for over a decade. Be it at a lecture, keynote, conference, webinar or workshop, his ability to captivate and inspire his public makes him a versatile and sought-after speaker.

Driven by the desire to help people achieve their absolute best, Dr Brett shares his vast knowledge and fresh, relatable content through powerful storytelling and a good dose of humour. Drawing from 20+ years experience working with clients in his busy Sydney clinic as well as being across the latest research, he delivers insightful and practical information that is on point and on trend, inspiring audiences to take charge and take action.

To find out more and book Brett to speak at your next event, either live or virtual, email hello@brettlillie.com

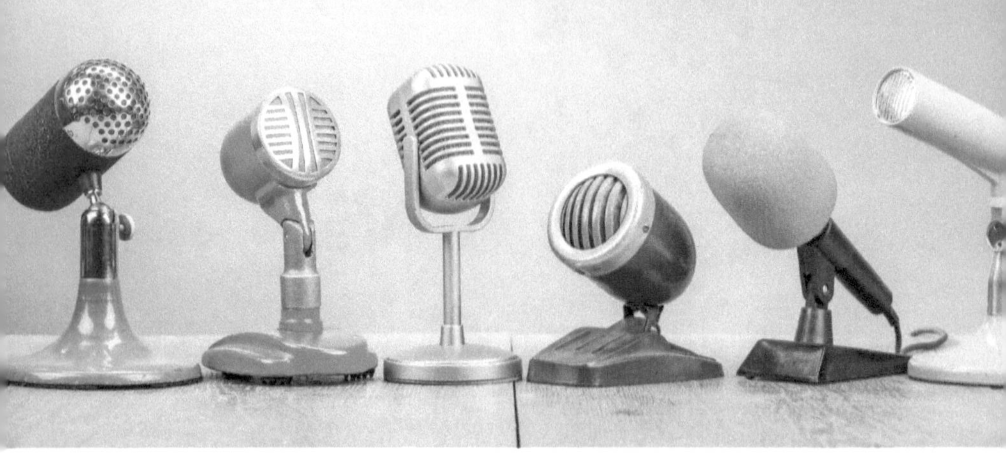

Would you like to interview Brett Lillie?

Dr Brett is a confident and engaging speaker and comfortable in all interview settings. He has great experience talking to the media. Camera crews have come to his clinic to showcase his work and ask his opinion on current matters.

Dr Brett can offer insights and talk about the following:

- Movement as the key to longevity

- Ageless performance

- From couch potato to inner athlete

- Improving and maintaining your energy

- Increasing productivity by thinking on your feet

- The modern epidemic called sedentary lifestyle

- The long-term effects of poor sleep

- Middle life crisis or golden years? Are you missing opportunities?

- The toll of stress and dealing with chronic pain

If you would like to interview Dr Brett about his book or any of the topics above, please email his team at hello@brettlillie.com

BIBLIOGRAPHY

Dyer, Prof. Wayne. 2010. *The Shift: Taking Your Life from Ambition to Meaning.* United States: Hay House

Grafton, Scott. 2020. *Physical Intelligence.* Great Britain: John Murray

Herman, Todd. 2019. *The Alter Ego.* New York: Harper Collins

Jha, Dr Amishi P. 2021. *Peak Mind.* Great Britain: Platkus

Keller, Gary. 2012. *The One Thing.* Austin, Texas: Bard Press

Mittleman, Stu. With Callan, Katherine. 2000. *Slow Burn.* New York: Harper Collins

Nestor, James. 2020. *Breath.* Great Britain: Penguin Random House UK

Panda, Sachin, PhD. 2018. *The Circadian Code.* New York: Rodale Books

Pontzer, Herman. 2021. *Burn.* Great Britain: Allen Lane

Robbins, Anthony. 2001. *Awaken The Giant Within.* United States: Simon & Schuster

Syed, Matthew. 2010. *Bounce.* London: Harper Collins

van der Kolk, Bessel. 2015. *The Body Keeps the Score.* Great Britain: Penguin Random House UK

Walker, Matthew. 2018. *Why We Sleep.* Great Britain: Penguin Random House UK

Zee, Prof. Phyllis C. *Sleep-Circadian Rhythms and Aging: A Bidirectional Relationship?.* Lecture, *Growth Sleep and Pain. What can go wrong? And what can we do about it?,* The American Academy of Craniofacial Pain Australian Chapter. Sydney March 19th-21st, 2021